W9-AFR-390

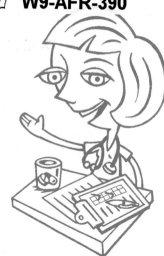

DATE DUE

1al-Newborn

Demystified

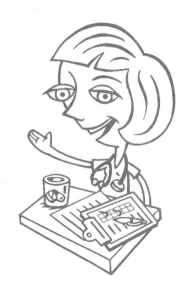

Maternal-Newborn Nursing Demystified

Joyce Y. Johnson, RN, PhD

Dean and Professor
College of Sciences and Health Professions
Albany State University
Albany, Georgia

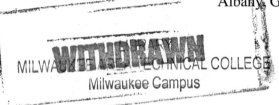
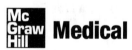

McGraw Hill **Medical**

**New York Chicago San Francisco Lisbon London
Madrid Mexico City Milan New Delhi San Juan
Seoul Singapore Sydney Toronto**

Maternal-Newborn Nursing Demystified

Copyright © 2010 by The McGraw-Hill Companies, Inc. All rights reserved. Printed in the United States of America. Except as permitted under the United States Copyright Act of 1976, no part of this publication may be reproduced or distributed in any form or by any means, or stored in a data base or retrieval system, without the prior written permission of the publisher.

1 2 3 4 5 6 7 8 9 0   DOC/DOC   14 13 12 11 10

ISBN 978-0-07-160914-2
MHID 0-07-160914-8

This book was set in Times Roman by Glyph International.
The editors were Joe Morita and Regina Y. Brown.
The production supervisor was Phil Galea.
Project management was provided by Gita Raman, Glyph International.
Cover design art directed by Margaret Webster-Shapiro.
The cover designer was Lance Lekander.
RR Donnelley was the printer and binder.

This book is printed on acid-free paper.

CIP data is on file with the Library of Congress.

McGraw-Hill books are available at special quantity discounts to use as premiums and sales promotions, or for use in corporate training programs. To contact a representative please e-mail us at bulksales@mcgraw-hill.com.

This book is dedicated to my mother Dorothy C. Young who has always been an inspiration to me, to my husband Larry, and to Virginia and Larry Jr. who are the wind beneath my wings. This book is also dedicated to our students who are the reason we teach and write. Much success in your nursing careers!

Joyce Y. Johnson

CONTRIBUTORS

Edna Boyd Davis, RN MN
Assistant Professor
Department of Nursing
Albany State University
Albany, Georgia
(*Chapter 12, Newborn Care*)

Cathy H. Williams, RN MSN DNP
Undergraduate Program Coordinator
Associate Professor
Department of Nursing
Albany State University
Albany, Georgia
(*Chapter 11, Postpartum Care*)

CONTENTS

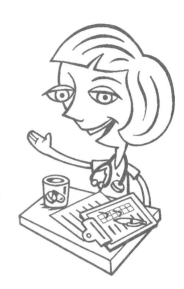

PREFACE

Maternal-Newborn Nursing Demystified is a detailed overview of the essential concepts involved in nursing care of the childbearing family with attention to the client. Because the childbearing process may involve the father and siblings in addition to the mother and newborn, nursing care should involve a family-centered process. Chapter 1 provides an overview of pregnancy, major terminology, and issues that may arise with young or older pregnant females. Chapter 2 focuses on family dynamics and community resources as well as issues related to cultural diversity. Chapter 3 focuses on the general health assessment that may impact the mother or newborn. Chapter 4 outlines contraception and discusses major problems that may occur prior to conception, including infertility and sexually transmitted disease. Chapters that address each stage of pregnancy and birth, in addition to the newborn period, follow with a systematic review of illnesses and conditions that may be encountered in each stage or period.

This book is an easy to understand presentation of concepts and focuses on the information that students most need to understand the conditions that most commonly face the childbearing family. This review focuses on the most critical information in maternal-newborn nursing by discussing the underlying factors involved in maintaining or restoring the health and well-being of the expectant mother and newborn, and those factors that threaten that well-being. *Maternal-Newborn Nursing Demystified* contains clear language and helpful features to guide the student through the application of concepts to real-life situations.

The book's features are organized as follows:

- Each detailed chapter contains objectives.
- Key terms are identified for the content area.
- A brief overview of the topic is provided.
- Content is divided into the following sections:
    - A brief review of anatomy and physiology, where applicable
    - Discussion of what went wrong that resulted in the condition
    - Signs and symptoms
    - Test results
    - Treatments
    - Nursing interventions

- Illustrations are provided to aid memory and understanding of the condition.
- Diagrams and tables are provided to summarize important details.
- Routine "checkups" are provided to briefly test understanding gained after a portion of the information is presented.
- A conclusion summarizes the content presented.
- A final "checkup" is provided with NCLEX-style questions to test the knowledge gained from the chapter.
- A comprehensive exam is provided, which includes NCLEX–style questions that cover content presented throughout the book.

Maternal-Newborn Nursing Demystified is a nursing student's best friend when studying for course exams and the NCLEX.

ACKNOWLEDGMENTS

I would like to thank Joe Morita for his direction and tremendous support in the development of this project.

Thank you to Edna Boyd Davis and Cathy Williams for their contributions to this project.

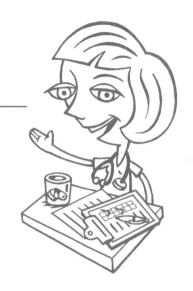

Roles and
Relationships

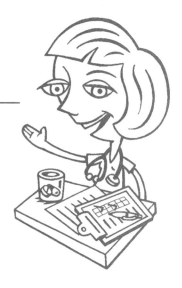

CHAPTER 1

Overview of Maternity Nursing

Objectives

At the end of this chapter the student will be able to:

1. Discuss the focus of maternal-newborn nursing.

2. Identify the varied roles a nurse may assume when caring for the childbearing family.

3. Discuss the steps of the nursing process in the care of the childbearing family.

4. Discuss the phases of maternal-newborn nursing.

5. Determine the impact of maternal growth and development stage on family planning and the care provided to the childbearing family.

 KEY TERMS

Antipartum phase
Certified nurse-midwife (CNM)
Clinical nurse specialist (CNS)
Family planning phase
Intrapartum phase

Licensed practical/licensed
  vocational nurse (LPN/LVN)
Nurse practioner (NP)
Puerperium

1 Maternal-newborn nursing focuses on the experience and care of a woman, family, and newborn before, during, and after a pregnancy. Care for the woman of childbearing age may begin prior to conception with planning for pregnancy and addressing issues related to fertility. A family-centered approach is essential to ensure that the primary needs of the childbearing woman and the newborn are fully addressed. The family provides the source of support and resources for the mother and child; thus the stability, or lack of stability, of the family can greatly impact the maternal-child experience before, during, and after pregnancy. The cultural background of the family also greatly impacts the experience of pregnancy and childbirth. Cultural norms should be respected and, when possible, integrated into the plan of care for the childbearing family.

The nurse's role in the care of the childbearing family can vary depending on the stage of the woman and family in the childbearing process. Prior to conception, the role of the nurse may be focused on assisting the woman and mate with family planning or addressing fertility issues. After conception and through delivery, the nurse is focused on supporting a healthy pregnancy through health promotion measures including proper nutrition, rest, and activity to benefit the mother and fetus. The nurse may work with the family in the following capacities.

- **2** **Licensed practical/licensed vocational nurse (LPN/LVN):** A technical nurse who has completed a program in a technical school or community college setting and passed the National Council Licensure Examination (NCLEX) for LPN/LVNs. The LPN/LVN may assist in a clinic, in a doctor's office, or in the hospital setting, often under the direction of a licensed registered nurse, nurse practitioner, or physician, and may assist with preparation of the childbearing female for the pregnancy and delivery process.
- **Registered nurse (RN):** A professional nurse who has graduated from an accredited nursing program and passed the NCLEX for RNs. The RN may plan and provide care for the childbearing family from initial contact, beginning with gathering of assessment data and providing teaching, to monitoring the progression of the pregnancy through delivery, and assisting the new family in the adjustment process with the newborn.
- **Nurse practioner (NP):** An advanced practice nurse who provides care to the childbearing family beginning with diagnosis and addressing of fertility issues with referral to appropriate specialists as needed, through delivery of the newborn and care of the neonate, and the postdelivery care for the new mother and family, including lactation guidance. The NP may specialize in women's health; family (FNP), focusing on all members of a family from birth to old age; the neonate (NNP), caring for the normal or high-risk newborn; or the pediatric client as the newborn grows (PNP).

- **Certified nurse-midwife (CNM):** An advanced practice nurse who is often educated at the master's level and has passed a certification test in the area of pregnancy and labor-delivery. The CNM provides care for the childbearing woman during pregnancy and through labor and delivery.
- **Clinical nurse specialist (CNS):** An RN who has obtained advanced education and clinical preparation at the master's level with a focus on the educator, manager, and researcher roles relative to patient care. The CNS may provide care to the childbearing family during the family planning phase, and through pregnancy and delivery, care of the newborn and postdelivery mother and family, and post discharge during the adjustment period with the newborn, including issues with lactation and refining parenting skills.

THE NURSING PROCESS

Nursing care is provided through the use of the nursing process, which provides a guide for comprehensive planning and provision of care to the childbearing family. After years of practice, the steps of the process might not be outlined distinctly as the nurse proceeds, but will remain the foundation for care. The process includes:

- Assessment of the client and family relative to the problem and related concerns, as well as underlying family dynamics that could impact support and resources needed during the childbearing process.
- Development of nursing diagnoses, which are statements that define the problems and potential problems indicated by the assessment findings. The North American Nurses Diagnosis Association International (NANDA-I: http://www.nanda.org) has established a list of standard diagnoses for use by nurses for planning and communication about client care.
- Determining the desired outcome of care and treatment—generally resolution, to the greatest degree possible, of the problem identified by the nursing diagnosis. Knowing the objective of the care, the desired outcome, helps to guide the activities needed and gives a basis for evaluating the success of the care.
- Nursing interventions designed to help the client and family meet the desired outcome of resolving the problem(s) from their condition. Interventions include care to the client as well as client and family teaching. Continued monitoring and assessment is also an expected nursing intervention for comprehensive client care.
- Evaluation, and revision as indicated. This is the final stage of the nursing process. Data are gathered and continued monitoring is used to determine the degree to which outcomes were met and the need to revise goals or interventions. New nursing diagnoses may be discovered, and old nursing diagnoses may be deleted after reviewing data from continued monitoring and evaluation.

4 Maternal-newborn nursing encompasses several phases:

○ **Family planning phase:** Involves the childbearing female from pubescence, with information on menstruation and avoidance of unwanted teen pregnancy, through addressing issues with infertility and preparation for conception and a health pregnancy

○ **Antipartum phase:** The period from conception until the beginning of labor

○ **Intrapartum phase:** The labor stages through the delivery of the newborn and placenta

○ **Postpartum phase (puerperium):** The stage after delivery of the placenta through 6 weeks following delivery

FAMILY PLANNING

The focus in family planning is to promote optimal well-being of the childbearing family including the health of the mother from conception through delivery, the safe and healthy delivery of a healthy newborn, or care of the high-risk newborn if indicated, and the establishment of a stable new family unit. Issues related to contraception, fertility, and other prepregnancy concerns are discussed in a later chapter.

The growth and development stage of the childbearing female greatly impacts the issues of conception being addressed in this stage. Of particular concern are pregnancy at a young age and pregnancy after the age of 40, both of which can increase the risk of complications.

CHILD OR ADOLESCENT PREGNANCY

Although the adolescent female is of childbearing age, the focus of nursing intervention at this time is frequently on prevention of unwanted pregnancy or comprehensive care in the case of teen pregnancy. Knowledge and consideration of a child's developmental stage can contribute to planning of age-appropriate care, particularly during pregnancy. Recognition that the stress of pregnancy can impact the child's growth and development allows the nurse to anticipate developmental disruption or regressions and plan care accordingly.

Potential Concerns

○ Risky behaviors, encouraged by peer pressure, i.e., violence, homicide, reckless driving, excessive and unprotected sexual intercourse, smoking, and substance abuse present a danger to the mother and fetus in child or adolescent pregnancy.

○ Mental health problems including depression, suicide, and eating disorders can lead to adolescent or fetal mortality or morbidity.

◐ Pregnancy can result in shame and decreased self-esteem due to feeling of being judged by adults and peers.

◐ Poor eating practices and decreased exercise contribute to malnourishment in the mother and fetus.

◐ Facial and body acne, aggravated by stress and hormones, is common in teens.

◐ Depression may be noted with higher levels in girls than boys:
  • Poor peer relations, depressed or emotionally unavailable parents, parental marital conflict or financial problems, family disruption through divorce, and poor self-image are contributing factors.

◐ Suicide ideation may manifest, particularly with fear related to parental reaction to pregnancy:
  • Preoccupation with themes of death
  • Talks of own death and desire to die
  • Loss of energy; exhaustion without cause
  • Flat affect; distant from others, social withdrawal
  • Antisocial or reckless behavior—alcohol, drugs, sexual promiscuity, fights
  • Change in appetite noted
  • Sleeping pattern changes noted, too little or too much
  • Decreased interest or decreased ability to concentrate
  • Gives away cherished items

Key issues in teen pregnancy include the following:
  • Emotional immaturity may decrease the teen's ability to cope with the responsibilities associated with pregnancy and motherhood.
  • Family support may be limited in unwanted pregnancy; this may be exacerbated by poverty or family dysfunction prior to the added stressor of teen pregnancy.
  • Nutritional needs are increased for the pregnant adolescent. Adolescent development is incomplete, resulting in a higher need for nutrients and a competition between the mother and infant often resulting in premature births, underweight newborns, malnourished mothers, and higher infant mortality:
    ◦ Maternal intake determines the adequacy of fetal nutrition and development. Deficits for the mother result in deficits for the fetus.
    ◦ Nutritional intake of the adolescent is frequently lacking in sufficient amounts of iron, calcium, and folic acid, which are highly important to developing muscles and bones and reproductive health.
    ◦ The teen diet is often deficient in vitamins A, D, B_{12} and zinc; thus vitamin supplements are critical for the pregnant adolescent.
    ◦ Nutrition counseling should involve the teen, the expectant father, and the families of the mother and father to ensure that proper nutrition is supported before and after the baby is born.

Nurse Alert **Teen nutritional intake is irregular; thus assessment of the teen's nutritional intake should be done over time and not involve just a 24-hour journal to determine eating habits.**

- Teen pregnancy may be associated with other high-risk adolescent behaviors such as drinking and drug use; thus a thorough assessment is needed and a plan of care should be developed to address any lifestyle habits that endanger the mother or fetus.
- Family dysfunction and abuse of the teen at home may place the adolescent mother at high risk for becoming an abusive parent or, at a minimum, establishing poor parenting skills.

Implications for Nursing Care

- Effective interventions for teen clients must involve the teen in the planning and implementation.
- All levels of development are important from physical to cognitive to psychosocial.
- Developmental stage theories are not specific for age, but include age ranges that may overlap.
- The stress of pregnancy and parenthood at a young age can cause reversal to a younger developmental stage for a brief period.
- Nursing measures, including client and family teaching, must consider the developmental stage the child is demonstrating.
- Teach adolescents and family members strategies to reduce health-compromising behaviors and address peer pressure.
- Monitor for signs and plan interventions to address depression and suicidal ideation.
- Relate health-enhancing behaviors, such as nutritious eating, regular exercise, and driving safety with use of seat belts, to improved physical appearance and promoting a healthy pregnancy and delivery.
- Assist the teen in planning an appropriate balance of activity and rest during pregnancy to minimize disruption of activities with peers.
- Provide opportunities for communication with the adolescent in the absence of parents to allow asking of personal questions.
- Daily hygiene and treatment with acne medication can reduce outbreaks, with caution to avoid any substances that may be harmful to the fetus.
- Age-appropriate care and teaching can reduce stress that the pregnant child or adolescent may experience during the growth and development process.
- Family interactions, or lack thereof, can impact growth and development and are particularly important to support a new adolescent mother in developing and sustaining good parenting skills.

PREGNANCY AFTER THE AGE OF 40

Increasing numbers of women, some of whom are career focused, are engaged in a second marriage, or have other life situations, decide to wait to conceive and have a child. Modern health care has greatly improved the outcomes for these women, with less mortality and morbidity resulting. However, pregnant women over the age of 40 may frequently be viewed as high risk, and may experience family disruption secondary to a mate who is unsupportive of the concept of childrearing in later life, or older children who are unprepared to share their parental support with a new sibling. Erikson's developmental stage of generativity versus self-absorption/stagnation indicates some behaviors that may be manifested by most women considering pregnancy or who are expectant mothers after the age of 40. For many women during this developmental stage career has been a major focus and may have been the reason for the delay in having children, but thoughts shift to caring for others and preparing the next generation. The woman and childbearing family must deal with conflicting demands, including fiscal needs for a two-person income or needs of aging parents. While focused on the pregnancy the woman may also feel the need to remain productive in her job, community, and other activities.

Key issues in pregnancy after the age of 40 include the following:

- Difficulty conceiving with increased risk of miscarriage or stillbirth
- Increased risk of complications during pregnancy, with higher risk in women with chronic illness or obesity
- Higher risk of developing diabetes secondary to pregnancy (gestational)
- Higher risk of pregnancy-induced hypertension
- Increased risk of developing preeclampsia (toxemia of pregnancy)
- Increased risk of requiring a caesarian section
- Increased risk of placenta previs
- Higher risk of delivering a child with a genetic/chromosomal abnormality, such as Down syndrome, possibly because the DNA in a woman's eggs is damaged over time (the risk rises as age increases)
- Developing a realistic plan for activity and rest during the pregnancy and balancing obligations during and after the adjustment period when mother and newborn are discharged home, which promote a healthy pregnancy and development of effective family management and parenting skills

Implications for Nursing Care

- Effective family planning is the first line of defense against potential problems. Educating the prospective mother/parents on the dangers of pregnancy after 40 increases awareness of possible complications and allows for preparation and informed choices.
- Assessment of the woman's preconception state allows for targeted efforts to improve health, prior to attempts to become pregnant.

- Harmful habits, such as smoking or substance abuse, including alcohol or nonprescription drugs, should be discontinued to provide the greatest chance of a healthy pregnancy.
- Obtaining optimal nutritional status and weight management is key to minimize the possible incidence of complications such as gestational diabetes or preeclampsia/toxemia.
- Blood testing for rubella titer and testing for other infections allow for early intervention to prevent fetal exposure to infections that could lead to miscarriage, stillbirth, or birth defects.
- Genetic counseling is beneficial to alert the prospective mother/parents of the risks of genetic abnormality related to older age. Family history should be examined to detect data that might indicate higher risk.
- Close monitoring after conception throughout the pregnancy allows for early detection of problems and early intervention to minimize harm to the fetus and protect the health of the mother.

ROUTINE CHECKUP

1. What is an accurate description of an advanced practice role in the care of the childbearing family?
   a. Licensed practical nurse
   b. Registered nurse
   c. Certified nurse-midwife
   d. Licensed vocational nurse

Answer:

2. Explain why adolescent pregnancy places the mother and child at risk for health problems.

Answer:

_____

_____

CONCLUSION

Factors related to family and community can positively or negatively impact the care of the childbearing family. The nurse should deliver family-centered care to ensure that support systems are maximized and not disrupted so that the childbearing family receives needed support prior to and throughout the pregnancy and through their return to the home and community. Several key points should be noted from this overview chapter:

1. Provision of family-centered care will require the use of an organized nursing process to gather assessment data and plan age-appropriate interventions for the childbearing family.
2. The nurse's role in the care of the childbearing family will vary based on the level of the nurse. The levels include licensed practical nurse, registered nurse, nurse practitioner (women's health, family, neonatal, or pediatric), certified nurse-midwife, or clinical nurse specialist.
3. Maternal-newborn nursing encompasses the family planning, antipartum, intrapartum, and postpartum/puerperium phases.
4. Family planning is focused on the optimal well-being of the childbearing family.
5. Performing family and community assessments is useful to identify contributing factors to possible problems with conception, support needed for the childbearing family, and risk factors for problems during pregnancy or after delivery. This assessment facilitates follow-up in the community or home setting after discharge.
6. Support the childbearing family with particular considerations for the adolescent or younger, or the older mother. If the mother is a child or adolescent, or is over the age of 40, complications may result that will impact the childbearing and childrearing process.
7. Nutritional assessment and support are important for a healthy pregnancy, particularly if the mother is a child or adolescent.
8. Pregnancy after 40 years of age can present physical and emotional challenges for the childbearing family.

? FINAL CHECKUP

1. **Which factors should be considered when a nurse assesses a pregnant client's growth and development? Select all that apply.**
   a. Food preferences
   b. Language skills
   c. Religious preference
   d. Changes in personality and emotions

2. **What is the major reason the family-centered approach is important when addressing the needs of the pregnant client?**
   a. Most insurance is acquired through a family plan.
   b. Pregnancy involves a mother, father, and child.
   c. A lack of family stability can impact the pregnancy experience for the mother and fetus.
   d. Most hospitals require that the family be included in the patient plan of care.

3. **What roles could a nurse assume in family planning?**
   a. Educator addressing issues of fertility
   b. Delivery room nurse
   c. Primary care provider
   d. a and b
   e. All of the above

4. **Which nurse could serve as a primary care provider for a pregnant woman?**
   a. Patricia, who is a licensed practical nurse
   b. Bryan, who is a registered nurse
   c. Lee, who is a certified nurse-midwife
   d. None of the above

5. **What would be the most appropriate desired outcome for a pregnant woman who is homeless and comes to the clinic for her first prenatal visit at 26 weeks gestation in a state of obvious malnutrition?**
   a. The woman will eat three nutritious meals each day.
   b. The woman will get a job and buy a home.
   c. The woman will give her baby to a family that can support it.
   d. The woman will return to the clinic on a weekly basis.

6. **The family planning phase would include what activities?**
   a. Delivering a healthy baby
   b. Discussing contraception
   c. Providing care during menopause
   d. All of the above

7. **Alecia is admitted to the clinic in active labor. She is in what phase of pregnancy?**
   a. Puerperium phase
   b. Intrapartum phase
   c. Antipartum phase
   d. Postpartum phase

8. **What is a major reason that the developmental stage of an expectant female could have an impact on the pregnancy?**
   a. None, really. The fetal developmental stage is more important.
   b. If the female is still living at home, her mother can parent the newborn.
   c. The female who is an adolescent will have nutritional and emotional needs that may conflict with the needs of pregnancy.
   d. The older female has completed all of her developmental stages by the age of 40 and can focus more on the needs of a newborn.

9. Clara, age 14, is admitted for dehydration secondary to continued vomiting in her first trimester of pregnancy. The nurse notes that Clara has her teddy bear and clings to her mother's arm. What would be the most likely explanation for Clara's behavior?

   a. The stress of pregnancy has caused Clara to revert to a younger developmental stage.

   b. Clara's overprotective mother has spoiled Clara, which is why she is pregnant.

   c. The pregnancy has affected Clara's brain and caused her to become retarded.

   d. Clara is trying to deny that she is pregnant by acting like a baby herself.

10. Ellisha, age 13, is pregnant and is admitted after experiencing diarrhea for the past 4 days. She is sullen and speaks only when her mother pushes her to answer questions. What should the nurse keep in mind when assessing Ellisha?

   a. Ellisha likely has a communication deficit due to complications of pregnancy.

   b. Ellisha would be more responsive to the nurse if her mother were absent.

   c. Ellisha's behavior is not important since her chief complaint is diarrhea.

   d. Ellisha is an adolescent and may also be quiet and sullen when she is well.

ANSWERS

Routine Checkup

1. c

2. Adolescents are still undergoing physical and emotional development with demands for calories and nutrients that may compete with the needs of the fetus and decreased coping mechanisms for handling the stressors of pregnancy and parenthood. The nutritional intake of a teen is inconsistent, leading to possible nutritional deficit and premature birth or low-weight neonate.

Final Checkup

1. b and d	2. c	3. e	4. e
5. a	6. b	7. b	8. c
9. a	10. d		

CHAPTER 2

Families and Communities

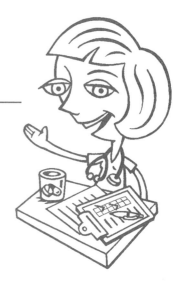

Objectives

At the end of this chapter the student will be able to:

1 Describe the impact of family dynamics on nursing care of the maternity client.

2 Distinguish the types of families in a community.

3 Contrast the health-related concerns for the childbearing family resulting from families and communities at varied socioeconomic levels.

4 Indicate appropriate nursing approaches to address family and community concerns related to the care of a family addressing pregnancy.

5 Discuss ethnic-cultural influences on family and community dynamics.

6 Determine appropriate nursing implications of ethnic-cultural concepts.

KEY TERMS

Assimilated family	Nuclear family
Cohabitation family	Reconstituted/binuclear family
Ethnocentric behavior	Sibling
Extended family	Stereotyping
Gay/lesbian family	Subculture
High-risk population	

OVERVIEW

The family and community greatly impact the experience stability of a childbearing family. Health promotion, maintenance, and restoration activities can be supported or hindered by family dynamics and the presence or absence of family and community support resources. Challenges presented by family or community distress can severely limit the stability of the childbearing family prior to, during, or after pregnancy and adjustment to parenthood. Understanding the basic concepts of family and community dynamics helps the nurse to provide comprehensive care to a childbearing family.

- Foundational concepts
  - Family-centered nursing recognizes family support as a needed factor for stability in the childbearing family.
  - The family, in addition to the expectant mother, is supported throughout the childbearing experience.
  - Collaboration with family is facilitated throughout hospital, community, and home care.
  - Family advocacy includes enabling families to build on current strengths and helping them maintain a sense of control over their lives.
  - In the home setting, the nurse is a visitor and should respect the authority of the family.
  - Community support resources are crucial for childbearing families with special needs—teen pregnancy, late pregnancy, or pregnancy with complications such as an expectant mother with illness or disability.
- Roles and relationships
  - Family members often play more than one role in the family system. Family roles:
    - Include but are not restricted to parent (mother, father, stepmother, stepfather, foster parent), child, sibling, provider, homemaker, or caregiver.
    - Vary depending on type and structure of the family, including number and age of members and ethnic-cultural background.

○ May change as a result of the pregnancy or the changes in the needs of the expectant mother—the mother may be unable to work when her income is essential to pay family bills. Pregnancy can cause stress in a family and that stress can in turn result in the distress of mother and fetus.

TYPES OF FAMILIES

Types of families may be described in different ways and needs may vary based on family composition and function. The types of childbearing families may include:

- **Nuclear family:** Husband (usually the provider), wife (usually home-maker, though frequently works also), and child/children.
- **Reconstituted/binuclear/blended family:** Consists of a child or children and one parent in one home and another parent in a different home. A step-parent and step-siblings may be present in one or both homes, reconstituting two families into one and resulting in two blended nuclear families.
- **Cohabitation family:** Consists of a man and woman who live together with a child or children without being married.
- **Single-parent family:** Consists of a man or woman living with one or more children.
- **Gay/lesbian family:** Two men or two women who live together as parents to one or more biological or adopted children.
- **Extended family:** Multigenerational groups consisting of parents and children with other relatives, i.e., grandparents, aunts, uncles, cousins, grandchildren.

NURSING IMPLICATIONS

- Perform a family assessment to determine the presence or absence of support for the expectant mother and father during and after hospitalization.
- Identify and collaborate with key individuals within the family unit to promote restoration and maintenance of stability for the childbearing family after the mother and newborn are discharged home.
- Involve parents and family in care activities with the newborn to promote learning of after-discharge care.
- Assess the home environment and determine the presence of factors contributing to risk for the pregnant client or the newborn after discharge from the hospital.
- Collaborate with family members to minimize risk factors and prepare the home environment to meet the needs of the expectant mother prior to delivery and the mother and newborn following discharge.

◑ Develop an action plan that addresses the needs of the childbearing family from admission through discharge back into the community and home setting.

SOCIAL AND ECONOMIC FACTORS

3 Social factors such as living environment and community relationships, in addition to economic factors such as poverty, unemployment, or homelessness, can impact the health and stability of the childbearing family due to limited access to clean water, food, shelter, or health care. Some groups are considered **high-risk populations**—groups of people at higher risk for illness than the general population, due to social, economic, or cultural factors.

Key social factors to be aware of include the following:

◑ Poverty may limit access to healthy food, leading to nutritional deficits.
◑ Lack of access to health care decreases health promotion and maintenance and contributes to late diagnosis of illness and delayed treatment.
◑ Unemployment contributes to poverty and possible homelessness, increasing exposure to overcrowded shelters, dangerous situations, and illness that may threaten the mother and fetus or newborn.
◑ High-risk behaviors such as unprotected sex, drugs, and reckless driving can lead to infections, addiction, and injury that increase infant and maternal mortality and morbidity.
◑ Teen pregnancy can result in poor prenatal care, premature birth, and birth defects, as well as poor parenting, leading to physiologic and psychological damage to the pediatric client.
◑ Family disruption due to factors such as drug or alcohol abuse, mental illness, domestic violence, or divorce can destabilize the childbearing family, leading to distress.
◑ Community instability due to gang activity, crime, violence, high unemployment, and poverty can result in decreased available health resources.

4 NURSING IMPLICATIONS

◑ Perform a community assessment to identify contributing factors to teen pregnancy, or risk factors for complications of pregnancy, such as communicable diseases.
◑ Address community resource needs prior to discharge with follow-up in the community or home setting after discharge.
◑ Work collaboratively with community agencies to provide comprehensive care to the childbearing family and facilitate follow-up assessment and evaluations.

ROUTINE CHECKUP 1

1. Bonita, age 16, lives with her father and the father's male lover. What type of family does Bonita have?
   a. Nuclear
   b. Binuclear
   c. Gay
   d. Blended

Answer:

2. Explain why poverty might place family members at risk for health problems.

Answer:

DIVERSITY ISSUES

Diversity commonly relates to ethnic and cultural differences found in persons of varied races or religious beliefs. Knowledge of practices that are acceptable or preferred and those that are forbidden allows the nurse to plan care that is appropriate according to the client's ethnic and cultural background. The most effective process for determining appropriate care is to ask the client, family, or significant other about preferences and taboos. Many cultural preferences and rituals do not conflict with medical care or pose harm to the expectant mother or fetus; however, some natural supplements may interact with medications or diet. Support of cultural norms can result in increased comfort and decreased anxiety for the childbearing family.

Some principles that should be considered when providing care to the childbearing family from varied ethnic or cultural origin include the following:

- Cultural norms are communicated from generation to generation.
- Many cultures have strong beliefs related to conception, pregnancy, delivery, and postdelivery maternal and newborn care. These beliefs should be honored whenever possible if no harm to mother or newborn is present.
- Clients from families that have first- or second-generation members who immigrated from a different culture are more likely to adhere to cultural rituals, while clients born in the United States or immigrating early in childhood may be fully **assimilated** (acculturated), having adopted American customs, cultural norms, behaviors, and attitudes.

- For a **subculture,** a group within a culture that has different beliefs and values from that deemed typical for the culture, the nurse should note individualized preferences.
- **Stereotyping** is categorizing a group of people together, usually by race, rather than respecting individual characteristics.
- In some cultures, females should not be addressed directly but through the dominant male family member.
- Some cultures are matriarchal with the oldest female family member accepted as the decision maker.
- Older family members in some cultures are respected as the decision makers for the family.
- In some cultures, it is unacceptable to touch a woman without permission, and only contact necessary for examination should be performed.
- **Ethnocentric** behavior (belief that one's own culture is best) can block communication with a client and family by decreasing trust and comfort.
- Communication in the native tongue may be needed for full understanding of client concerns.

NURSING IMPLICATIONS

Consider the following concepts when providing care to clients from different ethnic-cultural groups:

Communication

- Assess the family interactions and relationships and consult with the expectant mother, family member (include the pregnant child or adolescent) to determine preference relative to communication and the decision-making process between nurse and family members.
- Nurses should monitor their own behavior and avoid imposing cultural preferences on the client.
- Provide an interpreter or use technology to assist in translation of concerns voiced in the client's native tongue.

Physical touch

- Determine taboos related to physical contact and, if possible, avoid unacceptable touching by asking the client or family to move the body part as the nurse performs the examination.
- When unacceptable touching is needed, explain the purpose and minimize contact as much as possible.
- Use a sheet to cover the body, exposing only those areas being examined, and preserve the patient's modesty during the examination.
- If cross-gender touch is forbidden and a male nurse is assigned to provide care, enlist a female assistant to provide physical care while the nurse manages care.

Diet and Rituals

- ◑ Ask the client and family about preferences because not all individuals from a cultural group practice the same rituals.
- ◑ Determine food preferences and relay information to a dietician to promote offering of appropriate meal choices.
- ◑ Instruct family regarding dietary restrictions and needs, when indicated, secondary to pregnancy and allow them to supply desired foods if otherwise unavailable.
- ◑ Instruct family to notify the nurse regarding any foods or supplements provided to the client to avoid harmful drug-substance interaction or harm to the fetus.
- ◑ Consult family prior to removal of jewelry, bedside structures, or ointments from the client or the room to avoid disruption of religious or cultural ritual for luck or well-being.

ROUTINE CHECKUP 2

1. The basic concepts of family and community dynamics include which of the following?
   a. Family support as a needed constant
   b. Family roles restricted to mother and father
   c. Family advocacy that enables families to maintain a sense of control
   d. a and c only

Answer:

2. If a client is experiencing mild contractions and the male nurse needs to assess the progression of labor, what steps should the nurse take prior to beginning the examination? What explanation would the nurse need to provide about touching that is needed for proper assessment?

Answer:

_____

_____

CONCLUSION

Factors related to family and community can positively or negatively impact the care of the childbearing family. The nurse should deliver family-centered care to ensure that support systems are maximized and not disrupted so that the family receives needed support before and throughout the pregnancy, and through their return to the home and community. Several key points should be noted from this overview chapter:

- ◐ Assessment of family and community provides the nurse with a full picture of risks that threaten and benefits that are available to promote the health of the childbearing family.
- ◐ Collaboration with community resources is key to a successful transition from the hospital to the home or community setting, particularly for expectant mothers with special needs (teen or older mothers).
- ◐ Cultural and ethnic preferences should be considered and accommodated when possible.
- ◐ The nurse should not impose cultural norms and preferences on the clients.

? FINAL CHECKUP

1. **Felecia is 14 and pregnant. Her mother has no family to support her during Felecia's pregnancy. The nurse would speak with the social worker about services to support which type of family?**
   a. Nuclear
   b. Single parent
   c. Extended
   d. Reconstituted

2. **What type of community assessment is most important for the nurse to do to determine if Dawn, a 45-year-old who is blind, single, and pregnant, should be discharged home?**
   a. Home
   b. Church
   c. School
   d. All of the above

3. **Ifehi is a pregnant 22-year-old from Brazil. Her husband asked for a female nurse because females cannot be touched by males who are not family members. How should the nurse respond?**
   a. Tell the mother that Ifehi has to request a female nurse since she is an adolescent.
   b. Inform the physician of the request and wait for an order to schedule female nurses for Ifehi.
   c. Introduce the male staff nurses so that Ifehi and her husband can become accustomed to them.
   d. Adjust the assignments as much as possible to provide female nurses to care for Ifehi.

4. **What cultural religious ceremony could be accommodated without monitoring by the nurse?**
   a. Drinking of herbal teas by the client several times a day to restore balance
   b. Rubbing of a chemical ointment on the head and torso to drive away spirits
   c. Keeping a statue of the mystical god of health on the client's bedside table
   d. Cooling the room temperature to block hot illnesses from the body

5. **Which of the following factors can be hindered or supported by the presence or absence of community support services?**
   a. Health promotion
   b. Family growth and development
   c. Health restoration activities
   d. All the above

6. **The basic concepts of family and community dynamics include which of the following?**
   a. Family support as a needed constant
   b. Family roles restricted to mother and father
   c. Family advocacy that enables families to maintain a sense of control
   d. a and c only

7. **Which example represents a reconstituted family?**
   a. Judy and her mother and father live in Kansas in fall and Paris in summer.
   b. Peter and his mother live in one house and his father and stepmother live across town.
   c. Angela and her two fathers live in an apartment attached to her grandparents' home.
   d. b and c only

8. **Sally says she lives with her two mothers and her brothers. Her family is probably classified as which of the following?**
   a. Cohabited family
   b. Lesbian family
   c. Family
   d. None of the above

9. **Papa Estavez wants to take his pregnant wife back to Mexico for delivery since he feels it will be more beneficial to the mother and newborn. This attitude is a possible example of which of the following?**
   a. The need to bring in a translator
   b. Ethnocentric behavior
   c. Acculturated behavior
   d. Subcultural behavior

10. **Nurses should be aware of what factors when assessing clients of a different ethnic or cultural group from their own?**
    a. Communication dynamics
    b. Dietary restrictions
    c. Religious rituals and taboos
    d. All the above

ANSWERS

Routine Checkup 1
1. c
2. Poverty could lead to poor nutrition, malnourishment, possible homelessness, exposure to overcrowded shelters, decreased hygiene and increased infections, dangerous situations, decreased access to medical services, and illness due to lack of health maintenance activities such as immunizations or dental treatments.

Routine Checkup 2
1. d
2. Explain the examination to the client and the positioning and touch involved; arrange to have a female staff member or family member present during the examination. Ask if there are any concerns, and if the client asks for a female nurse, try to accommodate her wishes.

Final Checkup

1. b	2. a	3. d	4. c	5. d
6. d	7. b	8. b	9. b	10. d

REFERENCES

Ladewig P, London M, Davidson M. *Contemporary Maternal-Newborn Nursing Care*. 7th ed. New York: Pearson; 2010.

Santrock JW. *A Topical Approach to Life-Span Development*. Boston: McGraw; 2002.

Wisemann J, ed. *Registered Nurse Maternal Newborn Nursing Review Module*. Edition 7.1. Assessment Technologies Institute LLC. KS: Stillwell; 2007.

WEBSITE

Pregnancy Today. Healthy and safe pregnancy: Pregnancy after 40—special risks and some precautions to take. http://www.pregnancytoday.com/articles/life-circumstances-and-challenges-during-pregnancy/pregnancy-after-40-6175/. Accessed November 5, 2009.

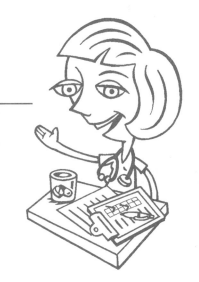

CHAPTER 3

Health Assessment of the Pediatric Client

Objectives

At the end of this chapter the student will be able to:

1. Discuss the role of communication skills in accurate assessment.

2. Determine assessment findings that deviate from the normal range for the maternal or newborn client.

3. Discuss the steps in assessment of family and community.

4. Distinguish diagnostic findings that indicate maternal or newborn health concerns.

5. Indicate appropriate nursing implications related to diagnostics and abnormal findings for the woman prior to, during, or after pregnancy, and for the newborn.

KEY TERMS

Abortion	Ecchymosis	Para
Blanching/capillary	Edema	Pectoriloquy
refill	Genu valgum	Petechiae
Body mass index/	Genu varum	Presumptive signs of
BMI	Gestation	pregnancy
Bronchophony	Gravida	Skin turgor
Chief complaint	Obesity	Stillbirth
Cyanosis	Overweight	Striae gravidarum

OVERVIEW

A comprehensive nursing history is one of the most crucial components in determining reproductive health. Health assessment provides key information needed for determining a client's condition and for planning of effective care to assist the mother and newborn. The nurse will move from assessing the client's and family's view of the pregnancy and any related problems through a client history, to assessing client support resources through a family/community assessment. The nurse will then proceed to the physical examination and review of diagnostic test results. Understanding the expected findings (normal ranges) for the maternal-newborn population will assist the nurse in detecting abnormal findings. Assessment is used in initial contact with the childbearing family and throughout the course of the plan of care to evaluate the health of the mother and child throughout the pregnancy and newborn period. Information found during the assessment is used to refine the plan of care to increase effectiveness and success in resolving or minimizing any problem(s) that occurs before, during, or after the pregnancy and newborn period. The nursing process, as discussed in Chapter 1, serves as a guide for assessment, planning, and delivery of comprehensive care to the childbearing family.

HEALTH ASSESSMENT: CLIENT HISTORY

COMMUNICATION

1 Communication is important when performing a health assessment. To provide family-centered care:

- All family members, including the father of the expected child and siblings, must be included in the assessment process because each perspective is needed to gather complete data on the mother and newborn's condition.

◐ Clear speech is necessary with the use of common terms instead of medical or nursing "jargon" that the client or family members may not understand.

Nurse Alert **If English is a second language for the client or family, an interpreter may be needed to ensure that the questions asked and responses given are understood. Communication in the client's native tongue may be needed for full understanding of client concerns.**

 Key considerations when communicating during a health assessment include the following:

◐ By encouraging all family members to talk, nurses can identify information that affects all aspects of the expectant mother or the newborn's life.

◐ Interviewing both the expectant mother and father, and children, if applicable, involves more than just gathering facts; this initial contact establishes the nature of future contacts and begins the development of a trusting relationship with the nurse.

◐ If the expectant mother and father are underage, involving their parents is important to determine resources and support.

Nurse Alert **Legally an expectant mother, even if underage, has rights to privacy; thus, consent should be obtained prior to sharing any information about the expectant mother with her parents or the expectant father or other significant others.**

◐ Begin the interview with an introduction; explain the nurse's role and the purpose of the interview to establish a clear nurse-family relationship.

◐ Treat the expectant mother and father (in child/teen pregnancy include their parents) as partners equal to the nurse in the care process.

◐ When speaking with children in the family, use an interview process that is appropriate for the child's developmental stage, including:
  • Use play with dolls or puppets; role-playing may ease the anxiety of the interview process.
  • Get at eye level with children and actively engage them through play and verbal exchange.

Nurse Alert **Be aware of cultural variation in eye contact, as direct eye contact might be considered disrespectful or evil.**

- Treat the adolescent appropriately, neither as a child nor an adult. Find time without parents present to allow adolescents to ask questions or state concerns they may be embarrassed to discuss around parents.
- Touch is a powerful communication tool, especially for the infant who calms when cuddled or patted, or a parent who is distraught about a child's condition.

 Nurse Alert **Be aware of cultural variation in physical contact, particularly across genders, which might be considered inappropriate or taboo.**

- Provide an interpreter or use technology to assist in the translation of questions and of responses voiced in the client's native tongue.
- Remember that nonverbal communication is as important as verbal. Smiling and maintaining a pleasant facial expression reduces client and parent anxiety.
- Attitude is also important in establishing a trust relationship with the client.
- ➊ Maintaining a non-judgmental manner will help the expectant mother feel comfortable providing truthful information to the nurse.

NURSING HISTORY

Discuss or have the client complete a form containing the following information to provide contact data and clarify concerns:

Demographic data:
- Biographical information:
  - Name of mother and expectant father.
  - Marital status.
  - Age of both parents, or newborn age and term of pregnancy.
  - Address/phone number(s) and other contact information. Include demographic data on the expectant mother's parents with teen/adolescent pregnancy.
  - Race.
  - Occupation.
  - Economic status.
  - Education level (current grade and school for adolescent).
  - Living situation.
  - Religion.

Past history provides background for the problem and any additional problems that the mother or newborn may have experienced. This assessment should include acute or chronic conditions, as well as surgical procedures.

Family history of congenital conditions, chronic illness, mental illness, causes of death, and birth types:

Maternal:

- Blood type and Rh factor
- Gynecologic background:
  - Last Pap smear (any abnormal findings)
  - Age at menarche
  - Incidence of dysmenorrheal
  - Sexual history and sexually transmitted diseases (STDs)
  - Contraceptive history
  - Problems with infertility and resolutions (fertility treatment, if any)
- Past pregnancies:
  - **Gestation:** Number of weeks since the first day of the last menstrual period.
  - **Abortion:** Birth before 20 weeks gestation or birth of fetus less than 500 g.
  - **Gravida:** Number of pregnancies, primi (first), multi (second or subsequent) pregnancy.
  - **Para:** Birth after 20 weeks gestation (live or stillborn), null (no births after 20 weeks), primi (one), multi (two or more) births.
  - **Stillbirth:** Newborn born dead after 20 weeks gestation.
  - Include each child's name; age; gender; duration of each pregnancy; complications, if any; outcome (live birth, abortion, stillborn); and type of delivery (vaginal or cesarean section).
- Last menstrual period (LMP) is needed to determine term (completion of 37 weeks of gestation).

Newborn:

- Nature of pregnancy: Expected term date and date of birth (preterm or post-term birth), maternal illness, substance abuse.
- Neonatal complications: In utero injury or infection exposure, birth defects, delivery trauma.
- Current state of health: For example, chronic illnesses, allergies, irritability, fatigue, amount of weight gain or loss, activity tolerance, abilities or disability in communication (nature of cry for newborn), mobility, pain or discomfort and source.
- Review of systems or head-to-toe approach should be used.
- **Chief Complaint:** Current symptoms determine why the expectant mother or newborn was brought in for examination (other than follow-up routine checkup).

2 Psychosocial:

- Sleep habits/sleep pattern: Difficulty sleeping or excess sleep is expected at different stages of pregnancy due to discomfort or fatigue, but it could indicate depression or drug reaction in some clients.

- ◑ Eating habits: Frequency and type of food intake can reveal inadequate diet or excessive intake, eating disorders, obesity, or malnutrition (failure to thrive in infant population), possibly due to poverty, or it could reveal abuse or neglect.
- ◑ Substance abuse: Drugs, tobacco, or alcohol (current or past) by expectant mother; determine frequency and amount or usage—could endanger the life of the mother and fetus and result in birth defects.
- ◑ Sexual activity and number of partners (do not limit assessment to older adolescents because a child as young as 8 or 9 may be sexually active): Increases risk of infections that may result in birth defects or premature birth.
- ◑ Expectant mother's (and father's, if available) acceptance and perspective on pregnancy: Determines if she is happy or distressed about the pregnancy.
- ◑ History of abuse (child abuse, spousal abuse).
- ◑ Plans for child post birth.

② NUTRITIONAL ASSESSMENT

An essential element in the assessment is an evaluation of the mother's or newborn's nutritional status from a physical examination and a biochemical perspective, as well as the usual dietary intake. It is important to collect data regarding nutrition habits.

- ◑ Inquire about community access to a variety of food types and factors impacting food choices, such as location of stores, fast-food choices due to time constraints, and economic barriers to purchase sufficient quantities of fresh fruits and vegetables and low-fat cuts of meat, as well as fish and fowl choices.
- ◑ If the family practices vegetarianism, inquire about the specific foods allowed and assess the adequacy of the intake of nutrients from all food groups.
- ◑ Assess whether the expectant mother is **overweight** (85–95% for body mass index [BMI]) or **obese** (weight above the 95% for BMI).
- ◑ Assess family members because family eating habits will play a large part in the eating habits of the expectant mother.

Nurse Alert **Assess dietary restrictions due to ethnic cultural beliefs and taboos.**

Nutritional assessment should include:
- ◑ Maternal dietary intake:
  - • Dietary history by 24-hour recall, food diary, or record to note the nature and amount of foods and beverages consumed (use longer assessment time for pregnant adolescent).

- Newborn dietary intake:
  - Determine if breast-fed and how often and how long the newborn feeds.
  - If newborn is bottle-fed or bottle supplements are provided, identify the type of formula and the amount of formula consumed and how often.
- Clinical examination:
  - Chart weight, height/length, and head circumference (for newborn) on a growth chart: If the newborn is below the 5th percentile (low birth weight) or above the 95th percentile, an insufficient or excess intake, respectively, is likely present.
  - Calculate **body mass index (BMI):** Weight in kilograms divided by height in meters^2.
  - Delay of development of **secondary sex characteristics** (i.e., breasts and pubic hair), which can indicate malnutrition, or vitamin A and D deficiency or excess.
  - Skin changes such as loss of **skin turgor** (elasticity of the skin) or **edema** (swelling or puffiness), indicating dehydration or fluid overload (preeclampsia).
  - Delayed wound healing (poor protein intake/malnutrition).
  - Flabby skin or stretch marks can indicate food excesses (other than that expected with pregnancy).

Other physical changes noting malnourishment or excess dietary intake should be included in the physical assessment.

BIOCHEMICAL TESTS

A general blood analysis of nutrients, electrolytes, and protein products should be performed.

- Hemoglobin and hematocrit: Low levels may reveal inadequate protein intake.
- Albumen, protein, creatinine, nitrogen: Low levels could indicate low protein intake.
- Glucose: Negative is normal in urine; blood glucose should be less than 100 mg.
- Tissue from hair, nails, bone, and organs can reveal nutritional deficits or excess chemical elements.
- Urinalysis can reveal excess glucose or other electrolytes, as well as protein loss from renal damage that could indicate a risk for protein deficit.

An economic assessment could indicate a financial deficit that limits the ability to buy food, indicating a need for assistance from social services.

FAMILY HISTORY AND REVIEW OF SYSTEMS

Questions about family history include items such as whether certain diseases/conditions run in the family, the age and cause of death for blood relatives (to detect possible genetic conditions), and family members with communicable diseases (to detect possible infection or infestation).

⬢ FAMILY ASSESSMENT

Family assessment is an important aspect of the history because the emotional and physical health of the child or adolescent is dependent on the stability of the family structure and function. There are various definitions for the term family, which broadly means one or more adults living with one or more children in a parent-child relationship. Family also refers to those individuals who are important to the core or nuclear group. Family assessment involves exploration of family structure and composition as well as member relationships, characteristics, interactions, and dynamics. If the expectant mother or father is experiencing a major stressor, such as parental divorce, chronic illness, or death of a family member, or issues such as behavioral or physical problems, or developmental delays that suggest family dysfunction are noted, an in-depth family assessment is indicated. In performing this assessment consider the following:
Structure:

- The number and composition of family members can determine the amount of support available to the child/adolescent during the health challenge.
- Questions should be open enough to encompass various family structures, such as, "What are the names of the newborn's parent(s)?" instead of asking about "husband or wife."
- Inquire about all persons living in the household or households in which the mother or newborn resides at any time, and their relationships to the mother/newborn and family, to provide a full picture of the family structure or multiple family structures the child is exposed to.
- Ask about extended family and additional support, such as from friends or church members, to determine the extent of resources available to the child and family.
- Inquire about family illness or deaths, previous separations, and divorces, and the child's response to these events to determine the use of previous coping skills.
- A genogram, a diagram of the family composition and structure, can be helpful in viewing the family structure comprehensively. The core unit is circled and connections of other members of the family to this core are clearly indicated (Fig. 3.1).

FAMILY FUNCTION

Family function assessment is focused on how members interact with one another. Several tests may be used to assess family function. A picture of the family from the child's perspective can be enlightening about the family relationships, as well as observation of the family interactions. The important aspects of this assessment are the determination of the family's ability to:

Sample genogram family

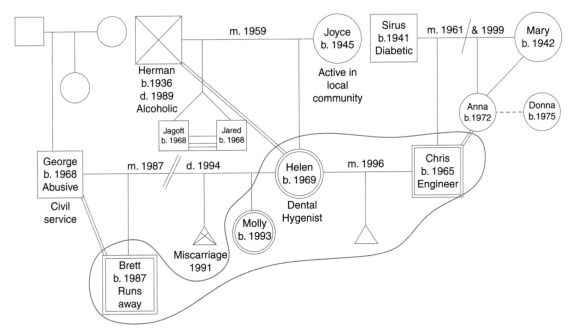

Figure 3.1 • Genogram.

◑ Adapt to stressors.
◑ Grow and mature.
◑ Work in partnership in decision making.
◑ Demonstrate affection and caring among the family members.
◑ Demonstrate resolve or commitment to assist family members.
◑ Perceive the value of time spent together and the importance of family time.

✔ ROUTINE CHECKUP 1

1. When performing a family assessment it is important to consider the _____ and the _____ of the mother's and newborn's family.

Answer:

2. Markie, a new mother at age 14, has a hearing deficit. Why would the nurse need to speak with the social worker about services to support Markie and her family?

Answer:

_____

_____

PHYSICAL EXAMINATION

A systematic approach to the physical examination, proceeding from head to toe, is the best method of fully assessing a client. For the newborn, however, intrusive procedures such as ear, eye, nose, and mouth examinations should be done last to keep the child calm for as long as possible during the physical examination. For the expectant mother, the examination of the abdominal area and uterus should be detailed to determine the progression of the pregnancy and possible complications. Normal findings for examination of most systems will vary for the expectant or postdelivery female depending on the stage of pregnancy or period postdelivery. Normal findings for the newborn will vary depending on time since birth and age (prematurity).

GENERAL

- ☾ Overall appearance reveals cleanliness, good nourishment.
- ☾ Mother's clothes are well-fitting, stature is appropriate for her age, posture is straight, no signs of pain (frown/grimace).
- ☾ Behavior and personality, interactions with significant others and nurse, **temperament** (behavioral style; calmness or lack thereof).

Nurse Alert **If the newborn is agitated, some assessments will need to be deferred until the newborn is more cooperative and calm to minimize distress.**

SKIN

- ☾ Integrity (absence of lesions, drainage, etc.).
- ☾ Color: **Pallor** (pale appearance) or **cyanosis** (bluish tinge) could indicate poor circulation or oxygenation; flushing could indicate increased blood flow to the skin due to infection.
- ☾ Texture, dryness or moisture, temperature, hair growth or lack thereof could indicate fluid or nutritional deficits.
- ☾ **Blanching/capillary refill** (pallor followed by return of flush after pressure; if this happens in less than 3 seconds it indicates circulatory adequacy).
- ☾ Birth-marks or other skin color deviations (non-pathological) may be noted.
- ☾ **Ecchymosis** (blue/black areas or bruises often from trauma) or abrasions (indicating trauma, accidental or intentional), or **petechiae**, small pinpoint hemorrhages, could indicate a bleeding disorder due to lack of platelets.

HAIR

- ☾ Note color, distribution, quality, texture, elasticity, and cleanliness. Cultural variations in coarseness or curliness of hair may be noted, but hair and scalp should be clean without lesions.

- Dry, thin, brittle hair, or hair loss can indicate nutritional deficits or be a side effect from medication/cancer treatment. Premature newborn may have thin hair over body (lanugo).
- Unusual hair distribution on face, arms, trunk, or legs could indicate pathology.
- Presence or absence of hair in underarm or pubic regions could indicate premature or delayed pubertal changes or hormonal dysfunction. Balding in an infant could suggest a need for more frequent position changes for sleep, although shedding of hair is expected for a newborn.
- Inspect for scalp itching, which could indicate seborrhea, ringworm, or scalp infection or infestation, i.e., lice (gray flakes from nits/ova adhering to hair, particularly in child/teen pregnancy due to exposure to other children).

Nurse alert **Use gloves or tongue blade during inspection for lice to avoid self-infestation. Also check scalp for ticks (smooth, oval, grey or brown bodies).**

NAILS

- Should be smooth and flexible.
- If dry and brittle, or ridges are noted, nutritional deficits may be present.
- Clubbed (bulged and slightly cyanotic) fingertips may indicate respiratory or cardiac dysfunction.

HEAD AND NECK

- Head control is absent in the newborn.
- Head shape and symmetry: Some **molding** (head is elongated due to overriding of head sutures) is noted after a vaginal birth. Report extreme asymmetry for further evaluation—flattening on one side could indicate lack of position changes.
- Fontanels should be open about 4–5 cm at the widest point (anterior) and 0.5–1 cm at the widest point (posterior). Report closed or narrow fontanels, or any pressure noted.
- Note reports of headaches, swollen neck glands, neck stiffness, or decreased range of motion.

Nurse alert **Nuchal rigidity—pain with neck flexion or hyperextension of head—may indicate meningeal irritation and possible meningitis (more common with adult than newborn).**

- Report any shift in trachea (possible lung problem), or mass in the neck.

EYES AND VISION

- Note size, symmetry, color, and movement of eyes, as well as exterior structures and spacing between the eyes; report deviations from expected straight palpebral fissures (upward slant normally noted in Asian clients). Down syndrome may be characterized by epicanthal folds, upward palpebral slant, and **hypertelorism** (large spacing between eyes).
- Eyelids should be smooth without drooping or malposition; note blink reflex.
- Examine pupil for roundness, equal size, reactivity to light, accommodation, and size, color, and clarity of iris (black and white speckling is seen in Down syndrome).
- The lens of the eye is normally not visible; white or gray spots could indicate cataracts.
- Report unusual eye movement, strabismus (often normal in newborn), excessively crossed eye.

EARS AND HEARING

- Inspect external ear structures for alignment, general hygiene, presence and amount of wax (can view partially without otoscope).
- Newborn may respond to human voice but should react to loud noise by demonstrating a startle (Moro) reflex and blink (acoustic) reflex.

Nurse Alert **Gently restrain newborn during otoscope use to avoid injury.**

- Pull pinna of the ear down and back for infants and up and back for adult to straighten the ear canal and visualize the inner ear structures.
- Auditory testing should be appropriate to age, ranging from a loud noise to elicit a startle reflex in the newborn to the use of audiometry for detection of the type and degree of hearing loss, if present in a child, adolescent, or adult.

MOUTH, THROAT, NOSE, SINUSES, AND NECK

- History can reveal high-risk circumstances: Frequent oral lesions, dental problems, or nosebleeds require in-depth examination of the mother.
- Report any flaring of the nostrils in newborn, which could indicate respiratory distress.
- Note any bleeding, swelling, discharge, dryness, or blockage of nasal passages, which could indicate trauma, irritation, or infection such as a cold.
- Mouth and throat may reveal lesions of the mouth or lips, redness, or drainage indicating infection. Congenital conditions such as cleft lip or palate may be noted.

- Fissures, stomatitis, or glossitis may indicate fluid and nutritional deficits.
- White patches in a newborn may indicate candidiasis, while herpes simplex or syphilitic chancre may be noted if the mother is an adult, adolescent, or child.
- Tonsil enlargement, redness, white patches, or drainage in the throat could indicate tonsillitis or pharyngitis.
- Inspect the teeth of the mother for dental caries, which could indicate poor hygiene and nutritional deficits, and also note malocclusion (poor biting relationship of teeth and poor tooth alignment), which could result in feeding problems, and loss of teeth and self-image problems.
- Palpate head and neck for lymph nodes and report swollen, tender, or warm nodes that may indicate the presence of infection.

CHEST

Heart, Neck Vessels, Pulses, and Blood Pressure

- Chest shape, symmetry, and movement should be noted. Report significant retraction of chest muscles, which could indicate respiratory distress.
- Note nipples for symmetry, discharge, masses, or lesions. Breast development usually occurs from 10–14 years, and engorgement is noted during pregnancy and the immediate postdelivery period, or beyond if breast-feeding.
- Listen to the heart with the mother in sitting and in supine position; note heart murmurs and record the location and volume intensity. Examine the newborn in supine position (an innocent murmur—systolic, short duration without transmission to other areas—may be noted in the newborn but should be recorded).
- Note history of congenital heart disease or hypertension.
- Neck vein distention could indicate congestive heart failure.
- Report if mother reports experiencing chest pain, or if newborn becomes fatigued or short of breath during feeding, as these are signs of decreased circulation or cardiac function.
- Resting pulse rates according to the age of the child:
  - Newborn: Pulse rate 100–160, up to 200 beats/minute if agitated
  - 10 years–adulthood: 55–90 beats/minute
- Blood pressure also varies according to age (systolic − age + 90/diastolic) but is rarely done in a well newborn. Average blood pressure for mother:
  - 11–18 years and older: 120/80 mm Hg

Lungs and Respiration

- Breath sounds should be clear; voice sounds should be heard through the lungs but syllables should be indistinct (vocal resonance). Syllables clearly heard when whispered (**pectoriloquy**), sound increased in intensity or clarity (bronchophony), diminished or absent vocal resonance, or decreased or absent breath sounds could indicate lung congestion or consolidation.

◑ Abnormal breath sounds should be described instead of labeled to promote diagnosis and monitoring by various health care providers. Breath sounds in the newborn may reveal hyper-resonance with loud and more intense sound since the chest wall is thin and sound is not muffled.

◑ Respiratory rates vary with age:
- <1 year: 30–35 breaths/minute
- 8–12 years: 19–20 breaths/minute
- 14–18 years and older: 16–18 breaths/minute

ABDOMEN

◑ Always auscultate before palpation or percussion of the abdomen to avoid altering current bowel sound pattern with artificial stimulation of bowel activity.

◑ Gently palpate abdomen; *do not* palpate abdomen if Wilms tumor is present.

◑ Note shape of abdomen: Newborn abdomen is prominent with umbilicus evident and moist initially—note color, moisture, and drainage, if present. Remnant of the umbilicus should be dry within days of birth.

◑ Examine all four quadrants of the abdomen.

◑ Report visible peristaltic waves, which may indicate pathologic state.

◑ Note absence of or asymmetrical abdominal reflex in newborn.

◑ Watch for increased intra-abdominal pressure from newborn cry and inspect for hernia in abdomen.

◑ Separation of abdominal muscle (**diastasis recti**) may be noted in the newborn due to immature muscles. Monitor for abdominal hernia (more common in African American newborn).

◑ Report hyperperistalsis, indicated by hyperactive bowel sounds, or an absence of bowel sounds, both of which may indicate a gastrointestinal disorder.

◑ Lack of tympany on percussion could indicate full stomach, or presence of fluid or solid tumor; avoid assessment of stomach immediately after meals.

◑ Note guarding and tenderness, particularly rebound tenderness or pain, which could indicate inflammation or infection.

GENITOURINARY

◑ Examination can be anxiety provoking for child and adolescent mothers; thus, secure privacy (ask mother's preference for parental or other significant other's presence), preserve modesty, and when possible offer same-sex examiner.

◑ If client complains of burning, frequency, or difficulty voiding, obtain urine specimen for possible culture.

○ Note urinary and genital structures, size, and appearance; explain anatomy for child who, though pregnant, may have no concept of her body. Caution that you will touch an area prior to doing so to prepare the client.

○ Expect that the testes will be undescended in newborns. Report urinary meatus that is not central at the tip of the shaft of the penis, large scrotal sac (possible hernia), or enlarged clitoris.

Nurse Alert **Female circumcision will produce a different genital appearance. Note and report the appearance but try not to react or show disapproval.**

○ Newborn genitalia may appear enlarged due to maternal hormone presence, which will subside over time.

○ If swelling, skin lesions, inflammation, drainage, or irregularities are noted, report for follow-up assessment for possible sexually transmitted disease (STD) or possible sexual abuse if an STD is noted in a young child.

○ Note any mass in the inguinal area that could indicate an inguinal hernia.

○ Anal protrusions, hemorrhoids, lesions, irritation, or mucosal tags should be noted and may require follow-up.

○ Diaper rash should be noted for treatment.

○ Perianal itching might indicate the need for testing for pinworms.

BACK AND EXTREMITIES

○ Note any lack or difficulty in mobility, or an uneven stance or gait, which might indicate uneven limbs or spinal curvature.

○ Waddle gait is often noted in late pregnancy as the mother compensates for the weight of the fetus, as well as backward bending of back to relieve pressure.

○ With child/adolescent standing erect and also with bending forward, note if curvature of the spine (**scoliosis**) is present and report for further examination if necessary.

○ Report rigidity in spinal column with movement from supine to sitting position, which might indicate a neurologic problem (i.e., meningitis).

○ Note joint mobility and presence of swelling, redness, warmth, or tenderness.

○ Ortolani's maneuver (have the client flex her knees while holding your thumbs mid-thigh and fingers over the trochanters, and abduct the legs and move the knees outward and down toward the table) may reveal congenital hip dysplasia. You may also use Barlow's maneuver (have the client flex her knees while holding your thumbs mid-thigh and fingers over the trochanters, and adduct the legs until your thumbs touch and feel for the head of the femur slipping out of the hip socket).

○ Bowlegs (**genu varum**) or knock-knees (**genu valgum**) that is asymmetric or extreme may indicate pathology and should be reported for further examination.

- Polydactyly (extra digits) or syndactyly (webbing) should be noted and reported.
- Muscle weakness or paresis (may indicate nutritional deficit), or extreme asymmetry of strength in extremities, hands, and fingers should be reported.

DEVELOPMENTAL MILESTONES

Developmental delays, detected through examination with tools such as the Denver II or other inventory, should be noted and reported along with any relevant historical data.

PHYSICAL MILESTONES

- Makes jerky, quivering arm thrusts
- Brings hands within range of eyes and mouth
- Moves head from side to side while lying on stomach
- Head flops backward if unsupported
- Keeps hands in tight fists
- Strong reflex movements
- Progresses from 5 to 8 feedings per day to 3 meals and 2 snacks by 12 months
- Progresses from sleeping 20 hours per day to 12 hours and 2 naps by 12 months

SENSORY MILESTONES

- Focuses 8–12 inches (20.3–30.4 cm) away.
- Eyes wander and occasionally cross.
- Prefers black-and-white or high-contrast patterns.
- Prefers the human face to all other patterns.
- Hearing is fully mature—recognizes some sounds.
- May turn toward familiar sounds and voices.
- Prefers sweet smells; avoids bitter or acidic smells.
- Prefers soft to coarse sensations.
- Dislikes rough or abrupt handling.

SOCIAL MILESTONES

- Birth to 1 month: helpless and dependent; makes eye contact but minimal social interaction; sleeps extensively

EMOTIONAL GROWTH

- Birth to 1 month: demonstrates general tension
- After 1 month: delight or distress shown

LANGUAGE DEVELOPMENT

Progresses from:

- ◐ Cries, grunts, and coos at birth to vocalizing in a controlled repetitive manner 'ma ma ma' or da da da' for example, by the age of 6 months; by one year of age progresses to simple sentences and 'conversation' with the 'adult' tone and manner of speech though some words are omitted.

ROUTINE CHECKUP 2

1. Current symptoms that determine why the child was brought in for treatment are called the_____ _____.

Answer:

2. Obesity is defined as being overweight. True or false?

Answer:

3. A bulging of the veins in the neck could indicate congestive heart failure. True or false?

Answer:

DIAGNOSTIC PROCEDURES

When preparing the client and family for diagnostic procedures, explain things as simply as possible and remain concrete and avoid abstractions. Be very clear about what the client needs to do (hold still, turn on side, etc.). Give the child/adolescent choices and control whenever possible in assisting during the diagnostic procedure.

◢ LABORATORY TESTS

Diagnostic findings, particularly biochemical tests, often vary based on the age of the client. The greatest age-related difference in test results is noted between those of the newborn and those of children above the age of 12 to adulthood. Lab values should be interpreted with consideration for client age. The following are examples of tests that may be performed:

Biochemical Tests

Pregnancy-specific tests may be performed from preconception tests to detect possible problems or complications to the pregnancy test.

- ◐ ABO blood typing and Rh factor determination (it's best for this to be done for both the expectant mother and father): If mother and fetus have different blood or Rh factor types a reaction can occur that can cause fetal and maternal death.
- ◐ First trimester aneuploidy screening: To detect abnormal chromosome condition.
- ◐ Serology test for syphilis to initiate treatment prior to conception if possible.

- Gonorrhea culture.
- Hepatitis B and HIV screening.
- Rubella titer: Hemagglutination-inhibition (HAI) test— 1:10 or above = immunity.

Blood analysis of nutrients, electrolytes, and protein products should be performed, as described in the earlier discussion of nutrition assessment. These and other tests can indicate dysfunction in the mother's or newborn's body systems.

- CBC (hematocrit, hemoglobin, red blood cell count, platelets): Decreased or increased levels may relate to respiratory, cardiovascular, renal, or bone marrow malfunction, or hydration problems (elevated hematocrit with hemoconcentration due to dehydration); decreased or elevated platelet levels can indicate risk for bleeding or clotting disorder.
- Prothrombin time (PT) or partial thromboplastin time (PTT): High levels mean blood is less likely to clot, indicating a risk for bleeding.
- Blood chemistries:
  - Potassium, sodium, chloride, calcium, magnesium, phosphorus, and others indicate electrolyte imbalances due to deficits or excess in dietary intake, malabsorption, or medication side effects, or glucose elevation or decrease (diabetes or pancreatitis).
  - Venous carbon dioxide, in addition to arterial blood gases, shows imbalances in respiratory system.
  - Blood urea nitrogen and creatinine reveal renal damage.
- White blood cell (WBC) count and erythrocyte sedimentation rate (ESR), which might be elevated in infection. WBC is decreased in bone marrow or immune system depression.
- Other serum/blood assessments specific to systems reveal adequacy or deficit in organ function. For example, AST, ALT (elevated in liver disease), HBeAg/HBsAg, IgM, IgG, anti-HBc (hepatitis B infection, current or past), anti-HCV, HCV RNA (hepatitis C), amylase and lipase (gastrointestinal function), T3, T4, TRH and TSH (elevated or depressed in thyroid disease), ACTH (pituitary function), or FSH, LH (gonad function).
- Peak or trough levels of medications (the highest or the lowest levels of a drug in the human system) may be drawn to guide treatments, elevations may result from renal malfunction or insufficient drug dosage.

Urine Testing

- Urinalysis may reveal decreased renal function or electrolyte imbalance such as excess glucose.
- Urine specific gravity may reveal low or high levels, which may relate to fluid depletion or overload.
- Pulse oximetry might be decreased due to respiratory abnormalities.
- Scope procedures: Direct visualization of body cavity to detect tumor, ulceration or irritation, or foreign body, and to obtain specimen

(biopsy)—bronchoscopy (lung blockage), gastroscopy (stomach irritation or blockage), colonoscopy (intestinal blockage or irritation), sigmoidoscopy (blockage).

- Scan or radioscope such as X-ray, magnetic resonance imaging (MRI), ultrasound, or sonogram: Allows for indirect view of deep body structures. Detects tumors, foreign bodies, narrowing of body passages, or openings between chambers (such as between heart chambers).

 Nurse Alert **Some procedures involve the use of contrast dyes to improve visualization of structures. Assess client for allergy to shellfish or iodine because the contrast can cause a severe allergic reaction (anaphylaxis) requiring life-saving measures.**

Nurse Alert **Determine if a woman is pregnant prior to X-ray and scans with dyes to prevent possible harm to fetus.**

- Electromyography (EMG), nerve conduction studies, or electroencephalogram (EEG) may indicate problems in nerve conduction in the brain or neuromuscular system.

NURSING IMPLICATIONS

The nurse should exercise caution during diagnostic procedures and data interpretation with pediatric clients.

- Explain that the smallest amount of blood possible is being taken from the newborn to reassure the mother and family.
- Warn the client that the needle injection will give a brief pain that will pass quickly.
- Store and label samples appropriately to avoid the need to repeat a test.
- Urine specimen collection may require attachment of a collection device to the perineum of a newborn or infant.
- Females in late pregnancy may need assistance in cleaning for a clean-catch urine specimen.
- Explain the procedure to the parent or family member who might assist the client if desired.

Nurse Alert **Be careful when interpreting lab values because the normal ranges of many lab values vary by age (newborn/infant, and 12 and older).**

ROUTINE CHECKUP 3

1. When performing physical assessments on newborns, intrusive procedures must be completed first to insure the accuracy of the assessment. True or false?

Answer:

2. Platelet deficits would most likely occur with what condition?
   a. Cardiovascular problems
   b. Bone marrow malfunction
   c. Diabetes
   d. Respiratory disorders

Answer:

3. When interpreting lab vales it is important to remember that "normal ranges" may vary by age. True or false?

Answer:

CONCLUSION

Factors related to family and community can positively or negatively impact the care of the childbearing family. The nurse should deliver family-centered care to ensure that support systems are maximized and not disrupted so that the client receives needed support throughout the illness and return to the home and community. Several key points should be noted from this overview chapter.

1. Provision of family-centered care will require the use of an organized nursing process to gather assessment data and plan age-appropriate interventions for the childbearing family.

2. Communication is critical to obtain information from and relay information to the childbearing family in the process of assessing and planning for client care; the family knows more about the client and their information should be valued.

3. Cultural and ethnic differences and preferences should be considered and accommodated when possible during the nursing care process.

4. History assessment is important to determine exposures and chronic conditions, as well as habits that may influence a client's health status.

5. Nutritional assessment and support is important to maintain and restore the health status of a child, adolescent, or adult going through pregnancy, or for the newborn.

6. Family assessment is important to determine support for the childbearing family during and after a pregnancy and adjustment to a newborn.

7. A physical examination should be performed systematically to determine symptoms of conditions that require treatment and that may impact

the pregnancy, delivery, and health of the mother and newborn.

8. Blood pressure, pulse, and respirations vary with age; consider normal based on the average value for age.

9. Assessment procedures may need to be altered depending on the age and condition of the client, such as light palpation only if a Wilms tumor is suspected, to avoid injury to the client.

10. Involve the client and family in the assessment and diagnostic procedures with a clear explanation of expected assistance.

11. Clearly explain what will be felt, seen, heard, or smelled by the client in preparation for a procedure.

12. Normal diagnostic findings and values should be interpreted based on the age of the client to determine what is truly abnormal.

13. Assess for pregnancy prior to X-ray or scans with dye.

14. Assess for allergy to seafood, shellfish, or iodine since some procedures may require contrast dye that contains iodine.

 FINAL CHECKUP

1. **What type of community assessment should be done to determine if Dawn, a pregnant 15-year-old who is blind after a recent accident, should be discharged home with a newborn?**
   a. Home
   b. Neighborhood
   c. School
   d. All of the above

2. **Iynuoma, a 21-year-old pregnant college student, has been admitted for observation. What are the key considerations for communicating during her health assessment?**
   a. Recognizing cultural differences and getting an interpreter if needed
   b. Asking close-ended, direct questions to establish trust
   c. Teaching Iynuoma and her family that the nurse is the expert in the care process
   d. a, b, and c

3. **Terri, who is 21 years old and homeless, is 4 months pregnant and has several small sores, sparse pubic hair, and a BMI under 65%. She is most likely suffering from which of the following?**
   a. Scoliosis
   b. Cyanosis
   c. Malnutrition
   d. None of the above

4. **Julie has low levels of hematocrit and albumen, as well as high levels of glucose in her urine. What are the possible implications of these symptoms?**
   a. A protein deficiency
   b. Renal damage
   c. A need for assistance from social services
   d. All the above

5. **At 36 weeks gestation, Susie has bruised areas on her arms, a light skin color with no red or pink undertones, and swelling in her feet and legs. Susie's symptoms can be described as which of the following?**
   a. Edema, pallor, and delayed development
   b. Pallor, hypertelorism, and petechiae
   c. Edema, ecchymosis, and pallor
   d. None of the above

6. **The number and composition of family members, instances of family illness or death, and parental divorce are all aspects of which of the following?**
   a. Temperament
   b. A client's family data
   c. a and b
   d. None the above

7. **Nuchal rigidity is described as which of the following?**
   a. A symptom of meningitis
   b. A symptom of cardiac dysfunction
   c. A headache symptom
   d. None of the above

8. **Hypertelorism is noted during the initial examination of a pregnant 13-year-old African-American female. She most likely suffers from which of the following?**
   a. Blindness
   b. Deafness
   c. Down syndrome
   d. None of the above

9. **White patches, redness, and excessive drainage are symptoms common to disorders of which of the following?**
   a. Ears and eyes
   b. Back and chest
   c. Skin and nails
   d. Mouth and throat

10. **The nurse involved in the health assessment of a pregnant client should remember which of the following?**
    a. Family and community can positively or negatively impact patient care.
    b. Cultural and ethnic preferences should be accommodated when possible to maximize success of patient care.
    c. Deliverance of family-centered care ensures that support systems are maximized and not disrupted.
    d. All the above.

ANSWERS

Routine Checkup 1
1. structure . . . function
2. An assessment of the family is needed to determine resources, and of the community to determine support needed (such as an educator who signs to communicate with the mother about parenting and infant care information).

Routine Checkup 2
1. chief complaints
2. False
3. True

Routine Checkup 3
1. False
2. b
3. True

Final Checkup

1. d	2. a	3. c	4. b	5. c
6. b	7. a	8. c	9. d	10. d

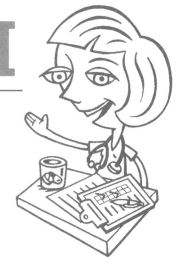

Systematic Exploration of Maternal-Newborn Conditions and Nursing Care

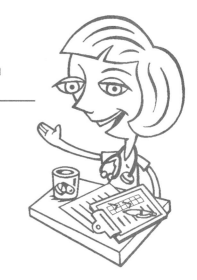

CHAPTER 4

Pre-pregnancy Preparation, Conception, and Genetic Considerations

Objectives

At the end of the chapter, the student will be able to:

1. Discuss the pre-pregnancy assessments and interventions needed to promote a healthy pregnancy and birth.

2. Identify conditions and circumstances that can prevent or complicate conception.

3. Discuss the process and periods of conception.

4. Evaluate diagnostic findings associated with congenital anomalies.

5 Discuss treatment regimens associated with congenital conditions.

6 Teach and support parents and families regarding the care required for a newborn with congenital conditions.

 KEY TERMS

Amnion	Genome
Carrier	Genotype
Chromosome	Phenotype
Conception	Recessive gene
Dominant gene	Teratogens
Embryo	Zygote
Fertilization	

OVERVIEW

The state of the mother and the father prior to the pregnancy can impact the pregnancy and the status of the unborn or newborn child.

PRE-PREGNANCY PREPARATION

1 Prior to pregnancy, the mother and father might be counseled to avoid lifestyle behaviors and exposure to circumstances or elements that might prevent pregnancy or result in harm or possibly death to the unborn child. Areas that should be considered include the following:

1.2 NUTRITION

- Malnutrition can inhibit menstruation, which can prevent pregnancy.
- A lack of folic acid in the maternal diet can lead to damage to the growing fetus, such as a neural tube defect like spina bifida.
- A paternal diet low in vitamin C has been associated with risk of birth defects and cancer.

2 AGE

As stated earlier, younger and older mothers may experience greater pregnancy difficulty or newborn complications.

- Increased infant mortality and premature births have been associated with adolescent pregnancy.
- Older paternal age has been associated with birth defects related to chromosomal damage, including Down syndrome.

SUBSTANCE ABUSE

- Nicotine: Smoking has been associated with low birth weight, as well as risk for cancer.
- Caffeine has been associated with low birth weight and preterm delivery.
- Alcohol: Excessive use of alcohol by the female during pregnancy can result in fetal alcohol syndrome (FAS), which includes facial, limb, and organ abnormalities, in addition to mental retardation. Additionally, moderate use of alcohol during pregnancy has been associated with decreased mental development in infants/children, adolescent alcohol use, and depression or anxiety as the child grows.
- Marijuana: Use by the father has been shown in some studies to reduce testosterone levels and sperm count, which may contribute to infertility. Use by the female has been associated with neurological damage resulting in tremors in newborns, and poor verbal skills and memory development.
- Cocaine: Use by the female could result in reduced birth weight and impaired mental and motor development, and use by the male may impact sperm and result in birth defects.
- Heroin: Use by the female can result in addiction of the infant and withdrawal symptoms including irritability, disturbed sleep, and poor motor control.

TOXIN EXPOSURE

- Some prescription and over-the-counter medications and other substances are **teratogens**—agents that cause fetal deformities and birth defects.
- Some teratogens are known and others are unknown; therefore, women of childbearing age who are attempting to become pregnant are encouraged to avoid medications without permission from their doctor, particularly during the first 3 months of pregnancy when development of body structures and organs are most sensitive to deformity.
- Maternal exposure to chemicals, radiation, pollutants, and toxic waste, including lead, mercury, or carbon monoxide, can result in visual, mental, or other defects. Exposure by a male to environmental hazards such as lead, radiation, pesticides, or other chemicals has been associated with abnormal sperm, which contributes to spontaneous abortion and conditions such as chromosomal abnormalities and childhood cancer.

Family planning includes instructing potential mothers and fathers to avoid habits that might reduce the chance of pregnancy or might result in damage to the infant or contribute to a difficult pregnancy.

CONCEPTION

To understand the complications that can occur before or during a pregnancy, the usual process of pregnancy from beginning to end should be understood. In order for pregnancy to occur, **ovulation**, the release of an egg from the woman's ovaries, must occur. Ovulation generally occurs 2 weeks before the menstrual period begins. The process of **conception** involves the union of a woman's ovum/egg with a man's sperm, also referred to as **fertilization**. Each parent contributes 23 chromosomes (genetic structures that contain information about characteristics) to the resulting child, who will have 23 pairs or a total of 46 chromosomes in each body cell. The genetic information in the chromosomes is found in a substance called deoxyribonucleic acid (DNA). The cells of the body are reproduced resulting in growth of the fertilized egg into a mass of cell. The fertilized egg is called a **zygote**, and the first 2 weeks after conception are called the germinal period, during which the cells continue to duplicate and move. This process begins in the woman's fallopian tube and the zygote moves to the uterus, where it implants into the uterine wall.

Two to eight weeks after conception, the embryonic period occurs in which:

- ◐ The cells of the zygote multiply and differentiate to form the tissues and organs of the body, becoming an **embryo**.
- ◐ The embryo's attachment to the uterine wall changes as layers, including the placenta, the umbilical cord, and the amnion, are formed.
- ◐ The placenta provides a mass of blood vessels from the mother and the embryo, across which oxygen and nutrients pass from the mother to the embryo and waste and carbon dioxide pass from the embryo to the mother.
- ◐ The umbilical cord, which contains 2 arteries and 1 vein, serves as a connection from the embryo to the placenta to allow blood flow from mother to child.
- ◐ The **amnion** is the sac in which the embryo will lie throughout the pregnancy. The fluid within the sac is produced by the embryo's kidneys, and as development continues this fluid is produced by the lungs as well.
- ◐ During the embryonic period, organ systems and body parts take shape.

3 The final period, the fetal period, begins 2 months after conception and continues through birth.

- ◐ The embryo is considered a fetus and proceeds to grow dynamically.
- ◐ Genitalia can be distinguished and gender can be identified.
- ◐ Increased movement of limbs and mouth is noted along with the gaining of length and weight.

TESTING

Pregnancy testing can be performed through blood or urine testing for the presence of human chorionic gonadotropin (hCG), a substance secreted during pregnancy. Blood testing is the most accurate and can assist in determining the duration of the pregnancy. The level of hCG increases each day of pregnancy; thus, the higher the amount of hCG, the longer the female has been pregnant. Blood testing is most often done in a laboratory facility.

Urine tests can be purchased and used in a home setting. These tests can be accurate; however, different products are sensitive to different levels (25 mIU/mL or higher) of hCG. In early pregnancy a test that is only sensitive to high levels of hCG might inaccurately indicate the woman is not pregnant when in fact the woman is. False-positive testing is less likely, unless medication being taken influences the test. If the test indicates the woman is pregnant, a follow-up test should be done in a doctor's office or other health care facility. Basic principles in pregnancy testing with urine include the following:

- Reading the instructions prior to testing
- Understanding the sensitivity of the test
- Using first morning urine or refraining from urinating for at least 4 hours prior to voiding for the test
- Avoiding drinking large amounts of fluid prior to testing since it can dilute the hCG in the urine and decrease test sensitivity to the hCG
- Reading the test package for medications that may impact the test results, and seeking medical testing for accuracy if indicated

Monitoring of hCG levels can indicate how well a pregnancy is progressing. If hCG levels are not increasing over time, the pregnancy might be endangered or have spontaneously terminated. Routine blood tests may be performed to determine the health of the mother, including blood levels through hematocrit and hemoglobin, electrolyte balance through potassium and sodium levels, or kidney function through blood urea nitrogen (BUN). If indicated, other system functions may be evaluated, such as blood gases if respiratory concerns arise.

ROUTINE CHECKUP 1

1. Why is it important for a woman to know she is pregnant as soon as possible after conception?

Answer:

_____

2. What period of pregnancy involves the initial development of buds that will later become extremities?
   a. Germinal period
   b. Fallopian period
   c. Fetal period
   d. Embryonic period

Answer:

3. What test result is most likely to be accurate?
   a. Negative urine test
   b. Negative blood test

Answer:

CONTRACEPTION

Understanding conception makes it easier to understand measures that can be taken to prevent pregnancy. Family planning involves the prevention of pregnancy until the desired time. Varied measures may be used to prevent fertilization of a woman's egg. Abstinence, or refraining from sexual intercourse, is the only 100% method of avoiding accidental pregnancy. Added benefits of abstinence include the decreased risk of sexually transmitted diseases (STDs). Other measures include nonprescription or prescription measures. Measures that involve barriers to sperm may also reduce the risk of STD transmission.

Nonprescriptive measures include measures to block the sperm from reaching the egg. These measures can include the following:

- Withdrawal of the penis prior to ejaculation to prevent introduction of sperm into the vagina. This measure has no cost; however, reliability is limited since leakage can occur prior to ejaculation being sensed by the male.
- Rhythm method, which involves abstaining from sex during times of fertility. This measure is inexpensive, but requires accurate monitoring of the menstrual cycle, which can be irregular in adolescence, making monitoring difficult.
- Condom to contain sperm (male) or block entry into the cervix (female) has low expense and provides protection against sexually transmitted disease, but may be difficult to apply (female). Condoms are readily available in stores but may be embarrassing to purchase, and condom breakage can occur.
- Spermicide: Serves as a chemical barrier to kill sperm prior to entry into the uterus. Spermicide is available in stores but may cause skin irritation.
- Diaphragm (a rubber cap lined with spermicide placed over the cervix) is used to block and kill sperm trying to enter the uterus. Use of a diaphragm may require a visit to a health care provider for fitting. The female must remember to apply it and must feel comfortable applying it before sexual intercourse. Use increases the risk of urinary tract infections and slippage of the diaphragm reduces effectiveness.

Some methods of contraception require a prescription and close monitoring to prevent complications. The risk of harm or injury must be compared with the benefit of pregnancy prevention prior to choosing to use these measures. Generally, the risk and expense are higher with prescription contraceptives. These measures may include the following:

- Oral contraceptive pill (OCP), or "the pill," which suppresses ovulation, alters cervical mucus, and thins the endometrial wall. The effectiveness is higher than nonprescription measures but hormonal changes can increase the risk of complications. This measure is expensive and requires medical monitoring; in addition, in some individuals "the pill" can increase the risk of cancer. Other risk factors for cancer, such as nicotine use, should be avoided if taking oral contraceptives.

○ Emergency contraceptive pill (ECP) can be administered up to 3 days after intercourse to stop implantation of a fertilized egg into the uterine wall.

○ Depo Provera injection of progestin only is given approximately every 3 months to suppress ovulation, thicken the mucus of the cervix, and thin the endometrial wall. It requires a health care provider visit. Complications may include weight gain, decreased libido, and decreased bone density.

○ Progestin and estrogen combination injection is provided monthly to prevent ovulation, thicken the mucus of the cervix, and thin the endometrial wall. It must be taken monthly, and nausea or tenderness of the breasts may be experienced.

Nurse Alert **History is critical with this therapy because if more than 33 days have lapsed since the last progestin and estrogen combination injection, a pregnancy test must be done prior to giving the injection to prevent unintended fetal damage in case of an unknown pregnancy.**

○ Norplant (levonorgestrel) implant is inserted beneath the skin of the upper arm to prevent ovulation, thicken cervical mucus, and thin the endometrial wall. Insertion and removal requires a medical visit, and it may be expensive to use. Weight gain may be noted with altered bleeding patterns.

○ Intrauterine device (IUD) blocks the sperm from contact with the egg and prevents implantation. If progestin is added, hormonal effects of thickening of the uterine wall and thinning of the endometrial wall are also noted. No systemic effects are noted, but the IUD may dislodge and be expelled; a medical visit is required. Irregular menstrual patterns may be noted with dysmenorrhea if the IUD is copper.

The choice of contraceptive requires client teaching and monitoring for complications, when indicated. Different methods may be used by a female or a male during their reproductive years. Some individuals have difficulty with fertility when contraceptives are discontinued. Thus, when couples plan to attempt pregnancy, they may transition to nonpharmacologic means of birth control for a period prior to discontinuing birth control entirely.

GENETIC CONSIDERATIONS

Many conditions can be transmitted from the parents to the infant through the genetic code passed along through the deoxyribonucleic acid (DNA). To evaluate the possibility of a child inheriting a condition, the genetic makeup of the parents is examined.

- The **genotype** is the gene/DNA composition of the individual.
- The **phenotype** is the expressed characteristics of the gene composition.
- Phenotypes may vary in nature and degree for persons of the same genotype.
- The most extreme manifestations of genetic genotype tend to occur least often.
- A **genome** is the set of instructions for the makeup of an individual. Studies have been done to map out human DNA to identify the source or marker for some conditions and behaviors with the hope of repairing or replacing defective genes with healthy ones.
- The importance of genetic testing of the parents is as follows:
  - It allows for the possibility of avoiding the transmission of defective genes through family planning with the choice not to reproduce.
  - It provides an opportunity for the parents to prepare for the birth of a child with a chromosomal abnormality.

4 Genetic conditions can be passed along through distinct mechanisms based on the dominant or recessive nature of the gene involved. Some conditions occur more often in persons who descended from certain geographic locations across the globe.

- A **dominant gene** exerts influence over another gene and thus the characteristic carried on the gene is expressed. For example, brown eye color may be on a dominant gene, and if a child has one gene with blue eye color and one with brown eye color, the child's eye color will be brown.
- Conversely, a **recessive gene** can only result in the expression of a characteristic if it is paired with another recessive gene for that characteristic. For example, if the gene for a disease is passed on in a recessive manner, both parents must provide the gene to the child in order for the child to manifest that disease.
- Individuals with one chromosome that has the condition and one that does not are considered "**carriers**," since they may not manifest any phenotype of the condition but are able to pass it along to their children.

Females carry two X chromosomes and males carry an X and a Y chromosome. Genetic traits and conditions might also be passed on through gender-linked genes.

- If a condition is linked to the X chromosome, the condition behaves as a recessive gene for the female who must have two genes that carry the condition in order to manifest it.
- The male will manifest the X-linked condition if his one X gene carries it because the Y gene carried by the male is unable to overcome the X gene.
- In order for a daughter to inherit an X-linked condition, the father must have the condition and the mother must either have the condition or be a carrier.

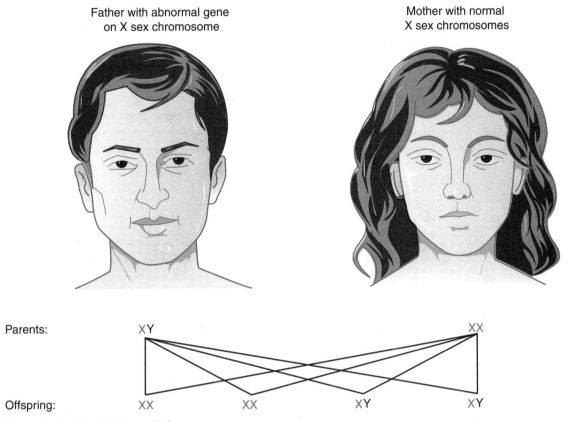

Figure 4.1 • Genetic transmission.

- The daughter of a father with an X-linked condition will at a minimum be a carrier since the X chromosome inherited from the father will be affected.
- A son can inherit a condition if the mother has the condition or is a carrier and passes the affected X chromosome to the son.
- The son of an affected father cannot inherit the condition if the mother does not have the condition and is not a carrier, because the son does not inherit the X chromosome from his father (Fig. 4.1).

SICKLE CELL ANEMIA

WHAT WENT WRONG?

In sickle cell anemia (SCA)/HgbSS cell disease, an abnormal gene results in production of an irregular red blood cell called hemoglobin (hgb) S, which replaces some of the normal hemoglobin A. The red blood cells collapse into a crescent shape (sickling) when stressed such as during dehydration, hypoxemia, or acidosis. When cells sickle, clumping is noted, which obstructs small blood vessels and blocks blood flow. These cells also have a short life span, resulting in early destruction due to damaged cell membranes and low blood count—anemia. This condition is an autosomal recessive condition requiring the gene from both parents. Some clients inherit one gene and may exhibit the sickle cell trait, which may or may not be symptomatic under severe conditions such as hypoxia during exertion in low oxygen settings (high altitude). Clients of African descent have a high incidence of sickle cell anemia.

Sickle cell anemia is a chronic illness with distress resulting from blocked and inadequate circulation and tissue/organ damage that causes pain and, over time, organ failure and death.

SIGNS AND SYMPTOMS

- Acute pain due to blocked blood vessels and tissue ischemia found in:
    - Extremities: Swelling of hands, feet, and joints—dactylitis (hand-foot syndrome)
    - Abdomen
    - Chest: Pain and pulmonary disease
    - Liver: Jaundice and hepatic coma
    - Kidney: Hematuria and impaired function
    - Brain: Stroke
    - Genitalia: Painful erection (priapism)
- Crisis episodes due to:
    - Vaso-occlusion: The most common crisis due to blocked blood flow from sickling
    - Sequestration
    - Aplastic crisis due to extreme drop in red blood cells (RBCs) (often viral trigger)
    - Megaloblastic anemia with excess need for folic acid or vitamin B_{12} resulting in deficiency
    - Hyperhemolytic crisis: Rapid RBC destruction—anemia, jaundice, and reticulocytosis
- Sickling episodes have exacerbation with remissions after effective treatment.
- Fatigue is secondary to the anemia.
- Fever during a sickling episode is possibly due to infection that provoked distress.
- Pooling of blood (sequestration) in organs resulting in enlargement:
    - Splenomegaly
    - Hepatomegaly
- Organ damage due to vessel blockage:
    - Heart (cardiomegaly) with weakened heart valves and heart murmur
    - Lungs, kidneys, liver, and spleen malfunction and failure

- Extremities: Avascular necrosis due to vascular blockage resulting in skeletal deformities (hip, shoulder, lordosis, and kyphosis) and possible osteomyelitis
- Central nervous system (seizures, paresis)
- Eyes: Visual disturbance, possible progressive retinal detachment and blindness
- Growth retardation may also be noted.

④ TEST RESULTS

- Low red blood cells (RBCs).
- Sickled cells noted per stained blood smear.
- Sickle-turbidity test (Sickledex).
- Hemoglobin, hematocrit, and platelets.
- Hemoglobin electrophoresis: Separation of blood into different hemoglobins to determine the form of hemoglobinopathies (hemoglobin defects).
- Newborn screening for SCA: Detects hemoglobin defects early.
- Pulse oximetry and blood gases may reveal hypoxia in severe anemia.
- Acidosis may result in a decreased serum pH level.
- Electrolyte imbalance may be noted due to acidosis.

⑤ TREATMENTS

- Hydration to thin blood and decrease sickling and vascular blockage.
- Minimize infection: Antibiotics may be ordered and vaccines recommended to avoid meningitis, pneumonia, and other infections.
- Oxygen supplement to decrease tissue ischemia.
- Pain medication: Oral or intravenous analgesics such as opioids.
- Electrolyte replacements may be ordered to correct imbalances.
- Blood replacement with packed cells if anemia is severe.
- Bed rest with mild range of motion during episodes.

NURSING INTERVENTION

- Pain control: Fear of addiction is not the issue during a crisis.
- Fluid intake: Monitor intravenous fluids closely to avoid fluid overload.
- Intake and output management to regulate volume and monitor kidney function.
- Rest periods during the day to avoid fatigue.
- Mild range of motion to retain mobility.

 ⑥ *Nurse Alert* **Avoid cold and cold compresses, which increase vasoconstriction and pain.**

Client and Family Teaching

❍ Teach proactive care to prevent episodes/crises:
- Get adequate fluid intake to prevent dehydration.
- Avoid infection or get early treatment for infection.
- Moderate activity and get adequate rest to avoid fatigue and hypoxia.

❍ Early signs of impending crisis: Splenic palpation to detect sequestration.

❍ Stress need for immediate care if there are signs of crisis.

❍ Genetic testing and counseling:
- Explain that SCA is an autosomal recessive condition requiring the gene from both parents.
- Encourage testing of siblings to allow for childbearing planning.
- Explain that each pregnancy when both parents are carriers presents a 25% chance a child will be born with the disease and a 50% chance the child will have the sickle cell trait.
- Refer for counseling and family planning if additional childbearing is desired.
- Discuss alternative parenting options: Insemination, adoption, etc.

❍ Support child and family with emotional responses, grieving, and coping:
- Allow ventilation of anger, concerns, fears, and questions.
- Provide support during depression over chronic illness.
- Provide honest responses regarding care during episodes.
- Use positive terms and avoid words like "crisis" when discussing vaso-occlusive or other problem episodes with the child and family.
- Encourage child to be in control of the condition and lifestyle needed to avoid episodes and promote maximum development.

✔ ROUTINE CHECKUP 2

1. Why should clients with sickle cell anemia be concerned if they marry a person with a sickle cell trait?

Answer:
_____
_____

2. What defect is most commonly caused by anemia?
   a. Increased red blood cell count and blood viscosity
   b. Depressed hematopoietic system and hyperactivity
   c. Increased presence of abnormal hemoglobin
   d. Decreased capacity of blood to carry oxygen

Answer:

HEMOPHILIA

Hemophilia is a group of congenital bleeding disorders due to a deficiency of specific coagulation proteins. This condition is occurs most commonly in persons of African descent, possibly as a genetic adaptation in trait carriers as protection from malaria.

WHAT WENT WRONG?

Hemophilia results most often from a genetic defect and most commonly a deficiency of factor VIII (hemophilia A) or factor IX (hemophilia B or Christmas disease). However, a third of hemophilia cases occur from a gene mutation. The X-linked form of the condition is passed when an affected male (XhY) mates with a female carrier (XhX) producing a 1 in 4 chance of the offspring having a girl or a boy with the disease, having a girl who is a carrier, or having a child without the disease or trait. The female carrier can also be symptomatic.

🔑 SIGNS AND SYMPTOMS

- Bleeding of varied degrees depending on the severity of the deficiency:
  - Spontaneous bleeding
  - Bleeding with trauma
  - Bleeding with major trauma or surgery
- **Hemarthrosis** (bleeding into the joints) in the knees, elbows, and ankles begins with stiffness, tingling, or ache as an early sign of bleeding and progressive damage.
- Warmth, redness, swelling, and severe pain, and loss of movement.
- Epistaxis (not the most frequent bleed).
- Hematomas may cause pain at the site due to pressure.
- Intracranial bleeding can cause changes in neurostatus and progress to death.

Nurse Alert **Bleeding from mouth, throat, or neck could result in airway obstruction and warrants immediate attention.**

🔑 TEST RESULTS

- History of bleeding with X-linked inheritance evidenced is diagnostic.
- Clotting factor function testing will reveal abnormalities in the ability to form fibrinogen or generate thromboplastin:
  - Whole blood clotting time
  - Prothrombin time (PT)
  - Partial thromboplastin time (PTT)
  - Thromboplastin generation test (TGT)

- Prothrombin consumption test
- Fibrinogen level

○ Pulse oximetry and blood gases may reveal hypoxia in severe anemia.

○ Acidosis may result in a decreased serum pH level.

○ Electrolyte imbalance may be noted due to acidosis.

5 TREATMENTS

○ Factor VIII concentrate to replace the missing clotting factor.

○ DDAVP (1-deamino-8-D-arginine vasopressin) for mild hemophilia (type I or IIA) to increase production of factor VIII.

○ Corticosteroids for chronic hemarthrosis, hematuria, or acute hemarthrosis.

○ Ibuprofen or other nonsteroidal anti-inflammatory drugs (NSAIDs) for pain relief.

Nurse Alert **NSAIDs should be used cautiously since they inhibit platelet function.**

○ Epsilon aminocaproic acid (EACA, Amicar) blocks clot destruction.
  - Exercise and physical therapy with active range of motion as client tolerates to strengthen muscles around joints.

Nurse Alert **After an acute episode avoid passive range of motion due to possible joint capsule stretching with bleeding. Client should control active range of motion according to pain tolerance.**

NURSING INTERVENTION

○ Maintain protective environment to prevent injury to client.

○ Monitor closely for signs of bleeding.

○ Treat bleeding episodes promptly.

○ Apply pressure to nares if nosebleed is noted.

○ Minimize crippling due to contractures and joint damage from bleeding:
  - Promote complete absorption of blood from joints.
  - Mild exercise of limbs during confinement to prevent disuse.
  - Encourage regular exercise regimen at home.

6 Client and Family Teaching

○ Protective care to prevent injury: Child-proof rooms with rounded corners, padding, etc., to minimize injury to mobile infant or toddler.

○ Non-contact sports and activities with minimum injury potential: Golf, swimming.

◐ Use safety equipment to minimize injury.

◐ Use a soft toothbrush with water irrigation for mouth care to prevent oral bleeding.

◐ Use an electric razor instead of blades for shaving.

◐ Teach to recognize a bleeding episode in the early stages and seek early treatment:

  • RICE: Rest, ice, compression, and elevation to control bleeding

◐ Wear a medical identification bracelet and notify the school nurse regarding the condition.

◐ Teach child to control the condition and lifestyle to avoid episodes and promote maximum development.

◐ Refer as needed for financial support if insurance ceases to cover client when over the age of 21 and removed from parent's insurance.

◐ Provide support for emotional stress to patient and family related to chronic condition.

◐ Genetic counseling:

  • Encourage testing of siblings to allow for childbearing planning.

  • Explain that for each pregnancy when father has the condition and the mother is a carrier there is a 50% chance that a female or male child will be born with the disease. There is a 100% chance a female child will have the trait for hemophilia if the father has the disease and the mother does not have the trait or the disease.

  • Refer for counseling and family planning if additional childbearing is desired.

  • Discuss alternative parenting options: Insemination, adoption, etc.

Nurse Alert **Avoid aspirin compounds and substitute acetaminophen since aspirin impairs platelet function.**

β-THALASSEMIA

Thalassemia is an inherited disorder involving deficiency in the production of globin chains in hemoglobin. The beta form of the disorder is the most common form and is found most often in persons of Greek, Italian, and Syrian descent. An alpha form of thalassemia is found in people of Chinese, Thai, African, and Mediterranean descent, possibly due to genetic mutation through intermarriages, or due to spontaneous mutation.

WHAT WENT WRONG?

Thalassemia is an autosomal recessive disorder in which the alpha or beta polypeptide chains in hemoglobin A are impacted. In β-thalassemia there is a decreased synthesis of the beta chains with an increased synthesis of alpha chains, resulting in defective hemoglobin and damaged red blood cells (hemolysis) and resulting anemia.

An overproduction of red blood cells (RBCs; immature cells) may result in compensation for the hemolysis. Folic acid deficiency may result from increased demand on bone marrow.

SIGNS AND SYMPTOMS

- Anemia with accompanying:
  - Pallor
  - Fatigue
  - Poor feeding
  - Progressive, chronic anemia: Hypoxia, headache, irritability, precordial and bone pain, and anorexia may be noted.
- Thalassemia minor occurs with a trait carrier condition and is non-symptomatic.
- Thalassemia intermedia manifests with splenomegaly and moderate to severe anemia.
- Thalassemia major (Cooley anemia) is severe anemia.
- Excessive iron storage in organs without organ damage (hemosiderosis) or with cellular damage (hemochromatosis) may be noted.
- Retarded growth, particularly delayed sexual maturation, is commonly noted.
- Bronzed complexion: Iron-containing pigment may be noted due to breakdown of RBCs and excess iron.
- If untreated, bone changes such as enlarged head and other facial changes may be noted.

TEST RESULTS

- RBC count is low.
- Hemoglobin and hematocrit levels are decreased.
- Hemoglobin electrophoresis analyzes the hemoglobin variants and helps in distinguishing the type and severity of thalassemia.

TREATMENTS

- Maintain adequate hemoglobin levels to reduce bony deformities and expansion of the bone marrow.
- Provide blood cells to promote growth and maintain activity tolerance:
  - Transfusions of RBCs as needed to keep hgb >9.5 g/dL
- Deferoxamine (Desferal), an iron-chelating agent, with oral vitamin C may be administered to promote iron excretion (may help growth if given early at 2–4 years of age).
- Bone marrow transplantation may be done in some children.
- Splenectomy may be done to decrease destruction of blood cells, if severe splenomegaly is noted.

Nurse Alert After splenectomy client is at risk for infection and should receive vaccines to prevent influenzae, meningitis, and pneumonia, in addition to regular immunizations.

NURSING INTERVENTION

- ◗ Promote adherence to treatment regimen.
- ◗ Support child during illness and distressing treatments.
- ◗ **6** Promote child and family coping:
    - Anticipate adolescent concerns related to appearance.
- ◗ Monitor closely for complications of the condition and treatment:
    - Multiple transfusions and iron buildup
    - Infection post-splenectomy
- ◗ **6** Genetic counseling:
    - Encourage testing of siblings to allow for childbearing planning.
    - Explain that for each pregnancy when both parents are carriers there is a 25% chance a child will be born with the disease and a 50% chance the child will have the thalassemia trait.
    - Refer for counseling and family planning if additional childbearing is desired.
    - Discuss alternative parenting options: Insemination, adoption, etc.

Some chromosomal abnormalities can occur if the 46 chromosomes do not divide evenly and one parent contributes an extra chromosome or a chromosome is missing. In most cases, infants will have a minimum of one X chromosome, but in some cases a male may have an extra X, giving a genotype of XXY instead of the XY. This condition is called Klinefelter syndrome and may be manifested with underdeveloped testes, enlarged breasts, and tall stature. Turner syndrome, on the other hand, is a condition in which females are missing an X chromosome, resulting in an XO instead of XX, or the second X is incomplete. The manifestations of this condition may include webbed neck, short stature, infertility, and difficulty with mathematics and possible problems with language.

A condition called fragile X syndrome is one in which the child receives a defective X, which often breaks. The primary manifestation is mental retardation, short attention span, and learning disability. These manifestations are more common in affected males since the female has an additional X chromosome that might block the defective gene's impact on the child.

DOWN SYNDROME

WHAT WENT WRONG?

Down syndrome is a genetic disorder resulting in retardation most commonly caused by 3 instead of 2 chromosomes 21. Down syndrome can also be caused by translocation of chromosome 21 where a portion breaks off and attaches to another chromosome.

Abnormal chromosomes might occur because the mother is older than 34 or the father is older than 41 at the time of conception. It might also occur because of a virus or radiation.

The degree of mental retardation will vary. Some patients are fully dependent on their caregivers. Other patients can function with little assistance.

SIGNS AND SYMPTOMS

- Broad, flat forehead
- Small oral cavity
- Protruding tongue
- Speckling of the irises (Brushfield's spots)
- Eyes slanting upward
- Low-set ears
- A single crease across the palm (simian crease)
- Hypotonia
- Mental retardation apparent in older infants

TEST RESULTS

- Pregnancy-associated plasma protein A serum test (PAPP-A): Performed during the first trimester to detect the level of plasma protein A that is covering the fertilized egg. A low level is linked to Down syndrome.
- Inhibit A serum test: Inhibit A inhibits the pituitary gland from producing the FSH hormone. An increased level of inhibit A is linked to Down syndrome.
- Human chorionic gonadotropin (hCG) hormone serum test: The placenta produces the human chorionic gonadotropin hormone, which is used to determine pregnancy. An increase in the β subunit of the human chorionic gonadotropin hormone is linked to Down syndrome.
- α-fetoprotein (AFP) serum test: A decrease in α-fetoprotein is linked to Down syndrome.
- Amniocentesis: Identifies the chromosome abnormality and is performed if the mother is older than 34 years of age or if the father carries a translocated chromosome.

TREATMENTS

- There is no cure for Down syndrome.
- Provide occupational therapy to help the child master the skills of independent living when possible.
- Provide speech therapy to help the child develop communications skills.
- Treatment is focused on treating the complications of Down syndrome such as trauma and infection.

NURSING INTERVENTION

- Explain the disorder to the family and suggest that they plan activities based on the child's abilities rather than the child's age, and involve the child in success-oriented activities.
- Maintain a routine to reduce the child's frustration.
- Arrange for a social worker to help the family deal with the challenges that face the child and the family.

✔ ROUTINE CHECKUP 3

1. A parent of a Down syndrome child calls saying that she has doubts about the diagnosis because her 2-month-old seems to act like her other child when she was 2 months old. What is the best response?
   a. "Call your health care provider and ask to have your child retested."
   b. "Your child has Down syndrome according to the child's test results."
   c. "Behavioral differences are not easily noticeable until later in the infant's development."
   d. "Your child has the facial characteristics of a child who has Down syndrome; therefore, your child has the disorder."

Answer:

CONCLUSION

The major principles in preparing for conception and pregnancy and using family planning and genetic testing include the following:

- Preparing for pregnancy requires guiding the prospective mothers or fathers toward decisions leading to optimal health status.
- Review of the process of conception makes it clear why early preparation of both the mother and father are important to promote a healthy pregnancy and birth.
- Family planning promotes the choice of the ideal time for a pregnancy.
- Understanding the process of conception helps in understanding the processes of contraception that will prevent or delay conception until the desired time:
  - Barrier protection blocks access of the sperm to the egg.
  - Several methods of barrier protection also protect against STDs.
  - Pharmacologic methods of contraception may prevent pregnancy but do not protect against STDs.
  - Choosing the best method for contraception requires weighing benefits against disadvantages.

○ Genetics can play a major part in decisions related to pregnancy and newborn care.

○ Genetic testing can reveal a high risk for fetal anomalies due to the transmission of conditions through dominant or recessive genes from the mother and father.

 FINAL CHECKUP

1. **What period of pregnancy involves the initial reproduction of cells that will later become the fetal body?**
   a. Germinal period
   b. Fallopian period
   c. Fetal period
   d. Embryonic period

2. **Which method of birth control will also provide some protection against sexually transmitted diseases?**
   a. Birth control pills
   b. IUD
   c. Condoms
   d. Abstinence
   e. c and d
   f. All of the above

3. **Which client would the nurse in a prenatal clinic need to see first?**
   a. M. Stevens, a 22-year-old in her first trimester who complains of nausea
   b. G. Dolyn, a 35-year-old in her second trimester who has urinary frequency
   c. L. Lyons, a 28-year-old who is pregnant for the second time and whose hCG level is the same this month as it was two months ago
   d. P. Joses, a 40-year-old who is at 36 weeks gestation and states she has felt the fetus move more than 15 times over the last 30 minutes

4. **The parents of a child with hemophilia are concerned about subsequent children having the disease. The mother is a carrier and the father does not have the disease. The nurse should know which of the following?**
   a. Hemophilia is not an inherited condition.
   b. All subsequent siblings will have hemophilia.
   c. Each sibling has a 25% chance of having hemophilia.
   d. There is a 50% chance of siblings having hemophilia.

5. A public health nurse is counseling a 38-year-old female client regarding birth control. The client has smoked since the age of 13 and sees "no need to quit now." Which type of birth control method would be *least* recommended by the nurse?
   a. Oral contraceptives
   b. Diaphragm
   c. Intrauterine device (IUD)
   d. Condoms

6. The symptoms noted in sickle cell anemia result primarily from which of the following?
   a. Decreased blood viscosity
   b. Deficiency in coagulation factor
   c. Increased blood cell destruction
   d. Decreased cell affinity for oxygen

7. Which statement best describes iron deficiency anemia in infants?
   a. Destruction of bone marrow and hematopoietic system depression is involved.
   b. It is easily diagnosed because of the infant's frail, emaciated appearance.
   c. It results from an inadequate intake of milk and the premature addition of solid foods.
   d. Decreased red blood cells leads to reduction in the amount of oxygen available to tissues.

8. The nurse should include what information when teaching the mother of an 8-month-old infant how to administer liquid iron preparations?
   a. Stop immediately if nausea and vomiting occur.
   b. Administer iron with meals to help absorption.
   c. Adequate dosage will turn the stools a tarry green color.
   d. Allow preparation to mix with saliva in mouth before swallowing.

9. In what condition is the normal adult hemoglobin partly or completely replaced by abnormal hemoglobin?
   a. Aplastic anemia
   b. Sickle cell anemia
   c. Iron deficiency anemia
   d. B_{12} deficiency anemia

10. What should be included in the plan of care for a preschool-age child who is admitted in a vaso-occlusive sickle cell crisis (pain episode)?
    a. Pain management
    b. Administration of heparin
    c. Factor VIII replacement
    d. Electrolyte replacement

ANSWERS

Routine Checkup 1

1. The woman needs to avoid agents that may cause developmental delays or fetal abnormalities during the early stages of growth when the fetus is most vulnerable.
2. d
3. b

Routine Checkup 2

1. If they have children, there is a 50% chance they will have a child with sickle cell disease.
2. a.

Routine Checkup 3

1. c

Final Checkup

1. a	2. e	3. c	4. c	5. a
6. c	7. d	8. c	9. b	10. a

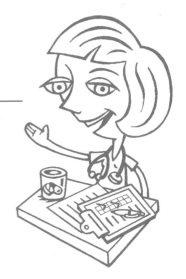

CHAPTER 5

Reproductive Health Issues

Objectives

At the end of this chapter, the student will be able to:

1. Discuss the risk factors for disruption of reproductive health.

2. Discuss signs and symptoms related to conditions that impact reproduction.

3. Evaluate diagnostic procedures associated with conditions that impact reproduction.

4. Discuss treatment regimens associated with conditions that impact reproduction.

5. Teach and support the client regarding prophylactic care and the treatment and care required for a family facing conditions that impact reproduction.

KEY TERMS

Abortion	Miscarriage
Aneuploidy	Missed abortion
Dyspareunia	Recurrent abortion
Hypospadias	Septic abortion
Incomplete abortion	Threatened abortion
Inevitable abortion	Varicocele
Infertility	Vas deferens

OVERVIEW

Pregnancy can present challenges to a childbearing family, but conditions encountered prior to pregnancy or in the early stages of pregnancy can pose a challenge to the pregnancy. Injury to, or infection of, reproductive structures could prevent or delay conception and pregnancy. Because fetal development in the early stages is sensitive to environmental factors, infection can result in congenital defects.

INFERTILITY

As stated in the previous chapter, conception requires fertilization of an ovum with a sperm. Pituitary hormones such as follicle-stimulating hormone (FSH) and luteinizing hormone (LH) are needed to stimulate the release of an egg from the ovaries. A pregnancy proceeds when the fertilized egg implants into the wall of the woman's uterus and the fetus grows until birth. Contraception can be used to prevent fertilization or pregnancy when desired, but sometimes fertilization or pregnancy is inhibited through unintended measures. The definition of **infertility** is the inability to become pregnant after 12 months of unprotected sexual intercourse. An expanded definition would include circumstances when a couple is unable to conceive or the woman is unable to carry a child to live birth, which both result in inability to bear a child. The causes of infertility are varied and the medical care required is specific to the teaching and interventions associated with the cause. Nursing care may include assisting with interventions or possibly supporting the couple if infertility cannot be resolved and they must seek alternative measures to having a child or resign themselves to remaining childless.

WHAT WENT WRONG?

Infertility can result from a number of causes, ranging from simple to complex. In order for fertilization to occur:

1. An egg must be released and travel into the fallopian tube.
2. Sufficient sperm must be released (ejaculated) into the vagina.
3. Sperm must swim through the uterus and enter the fallopian tube.
4. Sperm must meet and penetrate the egg.
5. The fertilized egg must travel down into the uterus.
6. The fertilized egg must implant in the uterine wall.

1 If anything goes wrong with any of these steps, secondary to the absence of eggs, blocked fallopian tubes, insufficient number or mobility of sperm, vaginal or uterine environment that is fatal to sperm, or uterine wall that is unreceptive to implantation, infertility can result.

2 SIGNS AND SYMPTOMS

- The primary symptom is inability to get pregnant after 1 year of trying.
- A woman may experience irregular or absent menstrual periods.
- Symptoms of hormone imbalance, including alterations in hair growth, sex organs, or sexual function, may be noted.
- If infertility is associated with an infection, vaginal or penile drainage and discomfort may be noted.
- Physical examination can reveal **hypospadias:** Urethral opening located on the underside of the penis preventing sperm from reaching the female cervix.

3 TEST RESULTS

- Physical examination:
  - Weight and height (obesity or anorexia can contribute to infertility).
  - Urethral opening located on the underside of the penis: **Hypospadias**.
- Ovulation testing: Blood testing for ovulation.
- FSH or LH levels may be too low to stimulate egg release.
- Hormone testing: Elevated prolactin or androgen levels (may block ovulation).
- Testosterone levels may be deficient.
- Hysterosalpingography (an X-ray to determine flow from uterus to fallopian tubes), or laparoscopy or culdoscopy (direct observation of the female pelvic organs) may reveal adhesions, altered ovaries that may impact function, or uterine anomalies (fibroid tumors).
- Pelvic ultrasound of the scrotum or uterus to determine structural defects or obstructions.
- Sperm analysis: Testing may reveal inadequate number or function.
  - Sperm count may be low (less than 5 million per mL of semen).
  - Sperm mobility may be limited.

- ◐ Endocervical culture may reveal an infection which may result in scarring of the fallopian tubes with blockage of the egg passage or that may present a danger to the mother and fetus.
- ◐ Male infection may impact sperm motility (prostatitis, epididymitis, or urethritis), sperm production (mumps), cause scarring with blockage of sperm passage
- ◐ Genetic testing may reveal a defect such as Klinefelter's syndrome (XXY chromosomes) in which the man has abnormal testicular development with absence of sperm production.
- ◐ Urinalysis may reveal sperm in urine, indicating retrograde ejaculation (backward flow).
- ◐ Nutrition testing for signs of malnutrition, particularly decreased vitamin B_{12}, iron, zinc, selenium, folate, and vitamin C.
- ◐ Steroid testing may reveal anabolic steroid levels that may cause testicles to shrink and decrease sperm production.
- ◐ Tests that reveal chronic illnesses that cause decreased sexual function such as cystic fibrosis (blocked **vas deferens**—the tube that carries sperm from the testes through the penis), diabetes (impotence, retrograde ejaculation), thyroid disease (hyper- or hypothyroidism can disrupt the menstrual cycle or cause impotence), anemia, HIV/AIDS, kidney disease, sickle cell disease (can contribute to fertility), or hypertension (medications can cause impotence).

④ TREATMENTS

- ◐ Early medical evaluation by a gynecologist if menstrual irregularity is noted, or a urologist if low sperm count or testicular, prostate, or sexual problems are noted, to promote early treatment.
- ◐ Increased sexual intercourse activity a minimum of 2–3 times per week may improve fertility. Refrain from ejaculation between intercourse activities.
- ◐ Proper nutrition with folate, zinc, and other nutrients, with limited caffeine and alcohol intake, which can increase risk of miscarriage.
- ◐ Avoid excessive exercise (8 hours or more per week), which can decrease ovulation.
- ◐ Smoking cessation, since tobacco can decrease fertility and contribute to miscarriage.
- ◐ Shield testes during cancer treatment with radiation, when possible, to prevent impairment of sperm production. Storage of sperm prior to treatment with chemotherapy or radiation may preserve sperm for later fertilization of egg.
- ◐ Surgical procedures to correct structural problems such as **varicocele** (mass of dilated veins within the scrotum that can elevate temperature and lower sperm count), hypospadias, or blocked vas deferens (fertility may be restored within 6 months to a year). A woman may undergo a salpingectomy to remove a damaged fallopian tube that might produce

fluid that is deadly to a zygote, or a scope procedure to remove mucous blockage of a fallopian tube.

- Clomiphene citrate may be administered to increase ovulation. Follicle development may be monitored with ultrasound, and intercourse or intrauterine insemination timed to promote fertilization.
- Intrauterine insemination may be performed if sperm are unable to penetrate the cervix due to mucus or other reasons.
- Human chorionic gonadotropin (hCG) may be administered by a fertility specialist to stimulate ovulation.
- In vitro fertilization—removal of eggs from the ovary, fertilization, then implantation of the fertilized egg into the uterus—and other high-tech treatments are well publicized but are used to treat less than 10% of all cases of infertility.

NURSING INTERVENTIONS

- Teach the couple the importance of proper diet and need for adequate folate, vitamins, and minerals to promote fertility and healthy pregnancy.
- Assist in screening of women for infections and pelvic inflammatory disease to promote early treatment.
- Emphasize the importance of the use of barriers to promote safe sex or the use of abstinence to avoid sexually transmitted diseases (STDs).
- Report findings from history and physical examination that may require treatment to promote fertility.
- Support female and male during fertility testing or in the decision not to undergo testing due to cost and discomfort.
- Assist the couple in withdrawal from abused substances including drugs, alcohol, smoking, and tobacco cessation as indicated.
- Instruct the couple on the importance of timing of fertility treatment and intercourse.
- Assist the couple in exploring alternatives including the use of a sperm or egg donor, surrogacy (use of another female to carry and deliver the child), or adoption.

Nurse Alert **Infertility issues can be sensitive for the couple involved; thus, the nurse must be non-judgmental and supportive of the couple's decision making.**

PREGNANCY TERMINATION

On some occasions an unintended pregnancy may occur, such as in adolescent pregnancy or in the case of rape. The female is faced with three alternatives: to complete the pregnancy and parent the child, to complete the pregnancy and allow the child to be adopted, or to terminate the pregnancy. Pregnancy can be terminated intentionally or can terminate spontaneously for a number of reasons. Pregnancy termination will be discussed from an intentional or a spontaneous perspective.

WHAT WENT WRONG?

An intentional or induced pregnancy termination (**abortion**) may be chosen when the pregnancy endangers the life of the mother, the fetus is at high risk of having a severe defect, or the pregnancy is undesired, possibly resulting from rape or abuse. In the case of adolescent pregnancy, the young woman may choose this option with or without her parent's input. Although abortion is a controversial issue, the health-care provider must remain objective and non-judgmental and allow the woman to make her own decision without being pressured.

Induced abortion can result in complications from retained products of conception such as the placenta, amnion, and fetus. Retained products can cause infection and eventual sepsis. Commonly septic abortion occurs with illegal abortions being performed by persons who have limited training or experience.

1 Spontaneous abortion/**miscarriage** is the death of the fetus or expelling of the fetus and placenta prior to the 20th week of pregnancy. An early miscarriage occurs before the 12th week and late miscarriage occurs between the 12th and 20th weeks of pregnancy. The most common causes of miscarriage include certain viruses—most notably herpes, parvovirus, cytomegalovirus, or the rubella virus—or conditions that prohibit normal development of the fetus, such as chromosomal anomalies. Trauma or immunologic anomalies can result in spontaneous abortion. Sometimes the cause is undetermined.

2 SIGNS AND SYMPTOMS

The symptoms of spontaneous abortion may vary depending on stage:

◑ Crampy pelvic pain, bleeding, and possible tissue expulsion. Abortion may present in varied forms:
  - **Threatened abortion** may present with vaginal bleeding (possible ruptured membrane) without cervical dilation.
  - **Inevitable abortion** may present with vaginal bleeding with cervical dilation (opening of cervical os will admit tip of finger).
  - **Incomplete abortion** will reveal expulsion of some products of conception (amnion, placenta, or fetus), and may appear like a blood clot; it could become septic due to remaining products.
  - **Septic abortion** will present with signs of infection including chills, pain, fever or hypothermia, vaginal discharge, and possible hypotension, oliguria, and respiratory distress from sepsis.
  - **Missed abortion** may have no symptoms immediately after fetal death due to the absence of bleeding or expulsion of product, but

growth of the fetus and fetal activity is not noted and over time may progress to septic abortion.
* **Recurrent abortion** occurs when two or more previous miscarriages were experienced.

❸ TEST RESULTS

- ◐ Urine test will be positive for hCG but without progressive increase in serum levels.
- ◐ Absent or low serum hCG could indicate abortion is complete, while higher levels could indicate incomplete abortion.
- ◐ Ultrasound will reveal an empty uterus or partial products of conception remaining in the uterus and absence of fetal heart beat in late abortion.
- ◐ Chromosomal assessment may be performed to determine if chromosomal abnormality such as **aneuploidy**—missing or extra X chromosome—may have contributed to the abortion (particularly in recurrent abortions).
- ◐ Endocrine disorders may reveal abnormal thyroid or glucose levels.
- ◐ Immune condition may reveal lupus or other antibodies.
- ◐ Physical examination may reveal incompetent cervix or structural anomaly in the cervix or uterus, such as polyps or fibroids, which may damage the fetus and result in abortion.

❹ TREATMENTS

- ◐ Bed rest to reduce cramping and bleeding.
- ◐ Abstain from sexual intercourse to prevent infection.
- ◐ Medical induction of labor and evacuation of products of conception may be performed for late abortion (16th week or later).
- ◐ Suction curettage may be performed to remove products of conception if earlier than 12th week of pregnancy.
- ◐ Partial or missed abortion (at 12th or later weeks) may require surgical scraping—dilation and curettage (D&C)—of the uterus to remove all products of conception.
- ◐ Administration of medication to cause cervical dilation to facilitate evacuation of the uterus may be done prior to D&C.
  * Antibiotics are administered for septic abortion.

❺ NURSING INTERVENTIONS

- ◐ Note women who are at risk for spontaneous abortion—particularly if previous miscarriages were experienced.
- ◐ If abortion is reported, monitor for signs of partially retained products of conception such as bleeding or signs of infection.
- ◐ Monitor for complications of uterine evacuation: Bleeding or uterine rupture, particularly in late abortion.

○ Provide emotional support in case of induced (intentional) or spontaneous abortion to assist female and male with feelings of guilt and grief.
Reassure female and male that spontaneous abortion is not due to actions
of either party.

○ In the case of induced abortion at the choice of the mother, remain supportive and non-judgmental, regardless of nurse's personal opinion.

○ If indicated, refer for counseling, particularly in the situation of recurrent
abortion.

SEXUALLY TRANSMITTED AND OTHER DISEASES

Sexually transmitted diseases (STDs) present a major danger to a female
prior to pregnancy, to an expectant mother, and to an unborn child. The incidence of STDs is high in adolescents and thus presents a particular risk factor
in adolescent pregnancy. Early diagnosis and treatment of an STD prior to pregnancy would be preferable, but treatment at as early a point as possible could
minimize the damage to the fetus and maternal morbidity or mortality. A group
of infections that can negatively affect the fetus during pregnancy is labeled
with the acronym TORCH, which represents Toxoplasmosis, Other infections,
Rubella (German measles), Cytomegalovirus, and Herpes simplex virus (HSV).

○ Toxoplasmosis is an infection contracted from eating uncooked or under-
cooked meat, or handling of cat stool. Symptoms are flu-like, or swollen
lymph nodes may be noted. Parasitic treatment is necessary with a combination of sulfadiazine and pyrimethamine, which could also harm the fetus.

○ Other infections include the sexually transmitted conditions discussed
later in this chapter.

○ Rubella is contracted from contact with children with German measles,
and the newborn may contract it from a mother who has rubella at the time
of birth. Symptoms for the woman include rash, mild lymphedema, muscle
aches, and joint pain, but fetal impact can include spontaneous abortion,
congenital abnormalities, and death. The primary intervention is prevention
with vaccination prior to pregnancy.

 Nurse Alert **Vaccination after pregnancy is contraindicated due to the risk of
contracting rubella.**

○ Cytomegalovirus is a herpes-related virus transmitted from contact with
the bodily fluids of an infected person. The fetus becomes infected in
utero or when passing through the birth canal if the mother is infected.
The woman is often asymptomatic and diagnosis by amniotic fluid culture is most reliable. Fetal impact can include growth restriction with
SGA (small-for-gestational age) infants, hydramnios, cardiomegaly, fetal

ascites, serious neurologic complications, or death due to tissue damage in utero.

- The herpes simplex virus is discussed later in the chapter.
- Because of the serious complications of the TORCH infections client education is crucial for women anticipating pregnancy. A screening is performed to identify these conditions in the mother or newborn at the earliest possible point.

CHLAMYDIAL INFECTION

WHAT WENT WRONG?

Chlamydia infection is caused by *Chlamydia trachomatis*, an organism that is partially parasitic and able to become part of the host cell despite the host's defenses. The organism then invades other host cells and within 40 hours manifests a full infection. Infections can progress to pelvic inflammatory disease (PID) and cause ectopic pregnancy, epididymitis, and infertility. The infection can also cause premature birth in addition to conjunctivitis and pneumonia in the newborn.

SIGNS AND SYMPTOMS

- Chlamydia may be asymptomatic for many infected with the organism.
- Vaginal discharge may be noted.
- Dysuria may be experienced by both males and females.
- Menstrual irregularities may occur if infection moves into the endometrium and fallopian tubes.
- Males may experience urethral discharge.
- Proctitis—inflammation of the anus and rectum—may be noted.

TEST RESULTS

- Culture from a urine, urethra, cervix, or vaginal specimen.
- Leukocyte esterase (LE) activity in urine is used to diagnose urethritis in males.
- Rapid antigen test, or polymerase or ligase chain reaction (PCR or LCR) tests.

TREATMENTS

- Azithromycin in a single dose.
- Doxycycline over 7 days.
- All sexual partners must be treated.
- Abstain from sexual intercourse until treatment is completed for both sexual partners to prevent reinfection.

NURSING INTERVENTIONS

- Instruct client on the importance of completing the full regimen of 7-day therapy.

○ Emphasize that failure to treat partners can result in repeat infection; thus, all partners should be treated.
○ Emphasize and explain the importance of abstaining from sexual intercourse until treatment is complete.

GONORRHEA

🔸 WHAT WENT WRONG?

This infection is caused by the bacteria *Neisseria gonorrhoeae*. The condition is often found in conjunction with a chlamydial infection and may be found after progression to PID. If infection occurs after the third month of pregnancy, the organism may be contained in the lower pelvic area in the urethra and cervix due to a mucous plug in the cervix that prevents expansion upward.

🔸 SIGNS AND SYMPTOMS

○ May be asymptomatic.
○ Common symptoms may be noted:
   • Greenish-yellow purulent vaginal discharge
   • Dysuria
   • Urinary frequency
○ Vulval inflammation.
○ Cervical swelling and erosion may be noted.

🔸 TEST RESULTS

○ Pre-pregnancy or initial prenatal screening (or end pregnancy testing for high-risk mothers) may reveal positive culture.
○ Urethral, throat, or rectal culture may be positive for gonorrhea if alternative entrance sites are used for sexual intercourse.

🔸 TREATMENTS

○ Non-pregnant women and partners may be treated with cefixime or ceftriaxone in combination with treatment for chlamydia with azithromycin or amoxicillin.
○ Cultures are repeated 1–2 weeks after treatment.
○ All sexual partners must be treated.
○ Pregnant women and partners must be treated with cefixime orally or ceftriaxone intramuscularly in combination with treatment for chlamydia with azithromycin or amoxicillin.

- Infected party should abstain from sexual intercourse until culture confirms that infection has been cured.

NURSING INTERVENTIONS

- Instruct client on the importance of completing the full regimen of antibiotic therapy.
- Emphasize that failure to treat partners can result in repeat infection; thus, all partners should be treated.
- Emphasize and explain the importance of abstaining from sexual intercourse until treatment is complete and culture confirms that infection is resolved.

PELVIC INFLAMMATORY DISEASE (PID)

WHAT WENT WRONG?

The infection of the endometrium, fallopian tubes, and the ovaries can be caused by several sexually transmitted organisms, including *N. gonorrhoeae*, *C. trachomatis*, or anaerobic bacteria. The spread of the infection can be fueled by the presence of an intrauterine device (IUD), douching, or menstruation, as well as active sperm, which can transmit the organisms into the genital tract.

SIGNS AND SYMPTOMS

- Tenderness in the lower abdomen and adnexal (tissue around the uterus) region.
- Fever (38.3°C [101°F] or higher).
- Cervical discharge and tenderness with movement.
- In adolescents, may manifest as generalized discomfort with lower abdominal pain and flu-like symptoms such as malaise, nausea, diarrhea, or constipation.
- Urinary tract symptoms.
- Infertility can occur due to scarring of the tubes.
- Ectopic pregnancy may occur after PID incident.
- Chronic abdominal pain.
- Abscess of the tubules and ovaries may be a complication.
- Fitz-Hugh-Curtis syndrome, with upper abdominal pain and possible peritoneal and hepatic adhesions.
- Prolonged pelvic pain or **dyspareunia** (painful sexual intercourse) may occur after PID.

TEST RESULTS

- Elevated erythrocyte sedimentation rate
- Elevated C-reactive protein
- Cultures positive for chlamydia or gonorrhea

TREATMENTS

- Cefoxitin or ceftriaxone intramuscularly in a single dose with doxycycline.
- Doxycycline twice a day over 14 days.
- If inpatient therapy needed (if pregnant adolescent or unable to tolerate outpatient care), intravenous antibiotics including gentamicin or clindamycin may be given.
- All sexual partners must be treated for infections to prevent recurrence.
- Abstain from sexual intercourse until treatment is complete for both partners.

NURSING INTERVENTIONS

- Teach the importance of using barrier precautions such as condoms to prevent the spread of STDs.
- Screen females and males for signs of infection to promote early treatment.
- Obtain specimen for culture and treatment.
- Encourage completion of full treatment of antibiotics to fully cure infection.
- Monitor closely for signs of ectopic pregnancy or other complications.
- Assist with pain management as indicated.

 # ROUTINE CHECKUP

1. Why is it critical to screen a woman for STDs prior to conception if she is interested in becoming pregnant?

Answer:

2. Women who test positive for chlamydia are often automatically treated for what other STD?
   a. Syphilis
   b. Herpes
   c. Human papillomavirus
   d. Gonorrhea

Answer:

HERPES GENITALIS

🔑 WHAT WENT WRONG?

Herpes infection involves the herpes simplex virus (HSV) and includes two forms: HSV-1 (oral-"cold sore") or HSV-2 (genital infection). The genital form is found in millions of people in the United States. The infection may remain dormant for periods of time with active occurrences triggered by stress, menstruation, pregnancy, vigorous intercourse, overheating, tight clothing, or exhaustion.

🔑 SIGNS AND SYMPTOMS

- Single or multiple vesicles noted in the anal, urethral, cervical, or vaginal areas appearing up to 20 days after exposure.
- Vesicles may rupture spontaneously and form painful, open, ulcerated lesions.
- Inflammation may cause urinary retention and painful urination.
- Inguinal lymph node enlargement may be noted.
- Flu-like symptoms.
- Genital pruritus.
- Lesions heal in 2 to 4 weeks.
- Less severe recurrences may be noted.
- Newborn injury or death can be caused by genital tract herpes during birth.

🔑 TEST RESULTS

- Culture of lesions will reveal the herpes virus.
- Polymerase chain reaction (PCR).
- Glycoprotein G-based type-specific assays.

🔑 TREATMENTS

- No known cure.
- Initial treatment with acyclovir, valacyclovir, or famciclovir.
- Suppression therapy may involve the above medications during recurrences.
- Pregnant women are provided acyclovir during the third trimester to reduce recurrences at time of birth.
- Povidone-iodine (Betadine) cleansing, vitamin C, or lysine may reduce recurrence.
- Burow's solution may reduce discomfort.
- Wearing loose clothing and cotton underwear promotes healing.

🔑 NURSING INTERVENTIONS

- Teach the importance of using barrier precautions such as condoms to prevent the spread of STDs.

- Screen females and males for signs of infection to promote early treatment.
- Obtain specimen for culture and treatment.
- Teach infected person to keep genital area clean and dry.
- Instruct on foods high in lysine and vitamin C.
- Stress the importance of preventing recurrence during birth.

SYPHILIS

1 WHAT WENT WRONG?

This chronic infection results from the spirochete *Treponema pallidum* acquired congenitally from the mother or through sexual intercourse with an infected individual or exposure to an open wound or infected blood. The infection occurs 10–90 days after exposure.

2 SIGNS AND SYMPTOMS

- No symptoms may be noted.
- Early stage may reveal a chancre at the entrance site of *T. pallidum*, which may be noted for 4 weeks.
- Fever, weight loss, and malaise may be noted.
- Secondary symptoms may be noted 6 weeks to 6 months after infection:
  - Condylomata lata (wart-like skin plaques/eruptions) on the vulva that are highly infectious
  - Acute arthritis, and liver and spleen enlargement
  - Non-tender, enlarged lymph nodes, and iritis
  - Chronic sore throat, and hoarseness
- Newborn may demonstrate secondary symptoms if infected in utero.
- If syphilis is transmitted transplacentally, intrauterine growth may be diminished.
- Preterm birth or stillbirth may be noted.

3 TEST RESULTS

- Prenatal serologic testing and third trimester testing may reveal syphilis (early testing may show a false negative).
- Dark-field examination may reveal spirochetes.
- Venereal disease research laboratory (VDRL) test, fluorescent treponemal antibody-absorption (FTA-ABS), or rapid plasma reagin (RPR) tests may be positive.

◢4 TREATMENTS

- ◐ Benzathine penicillin G is administered intramuscularly in a single dose if the person has been infected for less than 1 year.
- ◐ For infections of longer than 1 year, the dosage is repeated once weekly for 3 weeks. Tetracycline or doxycycline can be given if the person is allergic to penicillin (pregnant woman may need to be desensitized to penicillin and treated).

◢5 NURSING INTERVENTIONS

- ◐ Teach the importance of using barrier precautions such as condoms to prevent the spread of STDs.
- ◐ Screen females and males for signs of infection to promote early treatment.
- ◐ Obtain specimen for culture and treatment.
- ◐ Stress the importance of treating sexual partners and refraining from intercourse until treatment is complete.
- ◐ Inform the mother that serology testing may show positive findings for 8 months and newborn may show positive findings for 3 months.

CONCLUSION

Conception and pregnancy, though a natural process, can meet many obstacles, beginning with becoming pregnant when desired.

- ◐ The problem of infertility can have a solution that requires medical or psychological intervention to resolve, or a complex basis with no resolution.
- ◐ Alternatives in infertility situations should be explored and decisions respected.
- ◐ The nurse can play a vital role in teaching the prospective mother and father the importance of prevention of infections or early treatment to avoid infertility or harm to the female, male, or the fetus if pregnancy occurs.
- ◐ Infections present a major danger to the prospective parent and the unborn child. As a major contributor to infertility, the eradication of infection is crucial.
- ◐ The treatment of the woman and all sexual partners is important to prevent reinfection.
- ◐ Elimination of infectious organisms, such as those represented by the TORCH acronym, prevents fetal exposure during vulnerable periods that could result in developmental deformities, premature birth, or stillbirth.

? FINAL CHECKUP

1. **A nurse assesses a female client in an urgent care facility. The client states that she "is worried" because she had unprotected sex last night. Which is the best response by the nurse?**
   a. "You should have thought of this before you had sex. We could have helped you."
   b. "Don't worry. You probably aren't pregnant after one mistake."
   c. "If pregnancy is your concern, emergency contraception is an option we can discuss."
   d. "You are OK if your partner had a sexually transmitted disease; we can treat you."

2. **A woman enters the clinic and complains of a cramping pain with bleeding but denies that any clots or other substances have passed. She states that she uses contraception but has missed her menstrual cycle for the past 2 months and this does not seem like menstrual bleeding. Her serum hCG levels are elevated. What condition should the nurse suspect?**
   a. Missed abortion
   b. Partial abortion
   c. Septic abortion
   d. Incomplete abortion

3. **What test would a couple be likely to receive if repeat spontaneous abortions occur?**
   a. Chromosomal assessment
   b. Serum sodium level measurement
   c. Stress electrocardiography
   d. 24-hour fasting urinalysis

4. **Which client would the home health nurse see first?**
   a. A pregnant female who is at 16 weeks gestation who complains of urinary frequency
   b. A pregnant female who is at 12 weeks gestation and reports that her boyfriend was diagnosed with herpes
   c. A woman who is at 37 weeks gestation with her first child who reports that she started having labor pains a half an hour ago
   d. A woman who is at 24 weeks gestation who complains of indigestion and inability to sleep unless she turns on her side

5. **What nursing action would be appropriate if a woman has had a voluntary abortion and is hospitalized overnight for slight hypotension resolved with IV fluids?**
   a. Send the hospital minister in to assist the woman with her guilt.
   b. Plan time to remain available in the woman's room in case she wants to talk.
   c. Suggest that the woman ask to bury the fetal remains, which will allow her to grieve.
   d. All of the above.

6. **What patient teaching might help a woman in early pregnancy avoid fetal exposure to the TORCH infections?**
   a. Requesting an immunization to the German measles to avoid having rubella at the time of delivery.
   b. Restrict sexual contact to oral sex only if partner may have the cytomegalovirus.
   c. Avoid having sex when open sores are noted as protection against the herpes virus.
   d. Ask her family to clean the cat's litter box for the duration of the pregnancy.

7. **What information provided by the pregnant client would indicate that more patient teaching is needed?**
   a. She states she completed the full dose of azithromycin to treat chlamydia.
   b. She indicated her partner was also taking medication to treat the infection.
   c. She expresses relief that since both of them were on medication, it was safe to have sex again.
   d. She asks for a referral for her baby's father, who she may also occasionally have sex with.

8. **What should the nurse advise the woman with pelvic inflammatory disease (PID) to do for contraception?**
   a. Use an IUD so that the diaphragm can be avoided.
   b. Avoid using a condom because the latex can cause the inflammation to worsen.
   c. Stop taking the medications prescribed for gonorrhea until the PID subsides.
   d. Do not douche because this can spread the infection.

9. **A patient is admitted with an ectopic pregnancy. What condition in the patient's history would be most significant to confirming her diagnosis?**
   a. A history of a live birth 2 years ago.
   b. Recent recovery from pelvic inflammatory disease.
   c. Her desire to have a baby.
   d. The woman has no signs of pain or drainage from the vagina.

10. A woman who is found to be positive for gonorrhea will most likely be tested for what other condition?
    a. Herpes
    b. Cytomegalovirus
    c. Chlamydia
    d. Syphilis

ANSWERS

Routine Checkup
1. This allows for treatment as quickly as possible to avoid exposure of the embryo or fetus to infectious organisms that can cause defects in organ and limb growth.
2. d

Final Checkup

1. c	2. d	3. a	4. b	5. b
6. d	7. c	8. d	9. b	10. c

CHAPTER 6

Physiologic Changes of Pregnancy

Objectives

At the end of this chapter, the student will be able to:

1 Discuss the signs and symptoms of pregnancy.

2 Review the changes that occur during each trimester of pregnancy.

3 Discuss assessments and interventions for each trimester that are needed to promote a healthy pregnancy and birth.

4 Identify conditions and circumstances that can complicate each trimester of pregnancy.

5 Evaluate diagnostic findings associated with pregnancy.

6 Discuss care and treatment regimens associated with each trimester of pregnancy.

7 Teach and support parents and families regarding the care required in each trimester of pregnancy.

KEY TERMS

Amniocentesis	Hegar's sign
Ballottement	Positive signs
Braxton-Hicks contractions	Presumptive signs
Chadwick's sign	Probable signs
Epistaxis	Pseudoanemia
Goodell's sign	Quickening
Gravity	Trimester

OVERVIEW

The stages of pregnancy have designated periods during which fetal growth and maternal changes occur. Each of the major periods is referred to as a **trimester** (roughly one-third of the approximate 9 months of pregnancy). In Chapter 3 the stages of fetal development were reviewed. The first trimester of pregnancy will incorporate the ovum and embryo stages and beginning fetal stages of development. The second and third trimesters involve the remaining time in the fetal stage. This chapter reviews the maternal changes experienced as the pregnancy proceeds from the first to the third trimester and related nursing care needed to support a healthy pregnancy.

❷ FIRST TRIMESTER OF PREGNANCY

The first trimester involves the time period from conception and formation of the zygote (ovum stage) through the transition to an embryo (15th day to 8 weeks) and then a fetus (week 9 to 12 or 13). This period includes the discovery that a pregnancy is under way and moves through the point at which the gender of the fetus can be determined. Several signs and symptoms are noted during this period.

❶ SIGNS AND SYMPTOMS

○ **Presumptive signs:** Subjective symptoms or objective signs that might lead the woman to suspect she might be pregnant.

• Amenorrhea	• Uterine enlargement
• Nausea and vomiting	• Linea nigra
• Fatigue	• **Cholasma:** Darkening of skin on the face (mask of pregnancy)
• Urinary frequency	
• **Quickening:** Fluttering movement of fetus felt by woman (weeks 16–20 gestation)	• Striae gravidarum
	• Breast changes
	• Darkened areola

◑ **Probable signs:** Changes noted during an assessment that contribute to the suspicion of pregnancy. These changes result from physical changes in the uterus during early pregnancy.

- Abdominal enlargement related to changes in uterine size, shape, and position
- Cervical changes
- **Chadwick's sign:** Deep purple-blue colored vaginal lining due to increased blood vessels
- **Goodell's sign:** Softening of the cervix
- **Hegar's sign:** Softening and increased flexibility of the lower uterus

- **Ballottement:** Rebound of unengaged fetus
- Positive pregnancy test
- Palpable fetal outline
- **Braxton-Hicks contractions:** False uterine contraction that, unlike true labor, causes minimal pain and are irregular contractions

---

◑ **Positive signs:** Signs that can exclusively be explained by pregnancy.
Once the pregnancy is confirmed, the health-care provider will determine the expected delivery date. Two methods may be used to determine the delivery date:
- Nagele's rule: Starting with the first day of the last menstrual cycle, subtract 3 months, and add 7 days and 1 year.
- McDonald's method: Start with the measurement of uterine fundal height in centimeters from the symphysis pubis to the top of the uterine fundus (between 18 to 30 weeks gestation age). Gestational age is equal to the fundal height.

- Fetal heart tones
- Cervical changes
- **Chadwick's sign:** Deep purple-blue colored vaginal lining due to increased blood vessels
- **Goodell's sign:** Softening of the cervix
- **Hegar's sign:** Softening and increased flexibility of the lower uterus

- **Ballottement:** Rebound of unengaged fetus
- Positive pregnancy test
- Palpable fetal outline
- **Braxton-Hicks contractions:** False uterine contraction that, unlike true labor, causes minimal pain and are irregular contractions

PHYSIOLOGIC CHANGES OF PREGNANCY

1. Menstrual cycle stops (in early months spotting may be noted), and the uterus enlarges, alters in shape, and shifts in position.

2. Integumentary/skin changes occur due to hormones and stretch of skin as body enlarges during pregnancy (striae gravidarum/stretch marks). Many changes disappear after pregnancy (cholasma) but some remain (stretch marks). Increased secretion of sebum and skin oiliness may be noted, and palmar erythema (pink palms) or spider nevi (small red angiomas) may be noted on the face, neck, chest, arms, and legs due to increased estrogen levels with increased blood flow to tissues.

3. Nose, sinuses, mouth, and throat may reveal nasal stuffiness, gums may be swollen and bleeding, and nosebleeds (**epistaxis**) may be noted due to vascular congestion from estrogen, in addition to voice changes due to laryngeal swelling.

4. Blood volume increases, and heart rate as well as cardiac output increase to meet the mother and fetus's needs. Increased plasma volume results in a dilution of red blood cells and a **pseudoanemia** (a physiologic anemia in which the blood cells are not decreased but the plasma volume causes fewer cells per volume).

5. Respiratory workload is increased as oxygen needs increase for the mother to supply oxygen for herself and the child, and clear respiratory waste.

6. Breast changes due to estrogen and progesterone include increased sensation, breast and nipple enlargement, superficial vein engorgement, striae gravidarum, and hyperpigmentation of the nipple and areola.

7. Abdominal muscles and pelvic ligaments stretch with the enlarging uterus. Lower pelvic pain may be noted. Progesterone causes decreased smooth muscle relaxation with slower stomach emptying and reflux/heartburn, and decreased gastric motility resulting in constipation. Increased blood flow and constipation contribute to hemorrhoids (rectal varicose veins). Nausea and vomiting of the first trimester, due to shifts in hormones, is accompanied by hunger due to increased demands for nutrients. Pressure on the stomach and intestines as the fetus grows will increase dyspepsia, heartburn, and constipation. Carbohydrate metabolism is altered, leading to hypoglycemia in the first and second trimesters from increased tissue sensitivity to insulin and increased use of glucose and production of insulin from beta cell hypertrophy and hyperplasia. In the third trimester, hyperglycemia may result from decreased tissue sensitivity to insulin.

8. Urinary patterns may change due to increased blood volume, with circulation to kidneys. Urinary frequency may be noted with increased frequency as the growing fetus presses against the bladder.

9. Hearing may be diminished and earache may be perceived due to increased vascularity of the inner ear and blockage of the eustachian tube and feeling of fullness in the ears.

WHAT WENT WRONG?

Gestational Trophoblastic Disease

During the early stage of pregnancy, the first trimester, there are several complications that may occur, beginning with the pregnancy itself.

- In a condition called gestational trophoblastic disease the trophoblastic villi in the placenta begin to degenerate and become swollen and filled with fluid. The embryo does not develop beyond the cell duplication, becoming a mole-like mass with an appearance similar to grape clusters. The genetic material in the mass can be derived from paternal DNA or maternally and paternally.
- While some fetal material might be present in the mass, and human chorionic gonadotropin (hCG) levels are high, there is no growth, organ development, or activity. Life is not present.
- Women at high risk for the condition are those with low protein intake or age extremes (<18 years old or >35 years old).
- The condition is strongly associated with choriocarcinoma.
- Three complications that occur in early pregnancy, and are discussed in a later chapter, are as follows:
  - Spontaneous abortion, fetal death prior to 20 weeks gestation, secondary to chromosomal abnormalities or other developmental issues or trauma.
  - Ectopic pregnancy, pregnancy that occurs outside the uterus.
  - Hyperemesis gravidarum (HEG) is excessive vomiting due to hormones that may result in malnutrition, dehydration, and other problems.

Signs and Symptoms

- Gestational trophoblastic disease may be discovered with:
  - Vaginal bleeding around the 16th week that is either brown or bright red (scant or heavy)
  - Rapid uterine growth beyond normal expected pregnancy growth
  - hCG levels that are elevated, accompanied by severe nausea and vomiting (hyperemesis)
  - Ultrasound that reveals vesicular growths but no fetus
  - Urinalysis that may contain proteinuria
  - Clear vaginal drainage from vesicles
  - Pregnancy-induced hypertension (edema, hypertension, proteinuria) prior to the 20th week of gestation

⑤ TEST RESULTS IN EARLY PREGNANCY

- ◐ History: **Gravity** (number of pregnancies), term births (38 weeks or greater), preterm births (37 weeks or fewer), abortions/miscarriages, live children, para (birth after 20 weeks gestation, live or stillborn), family history, lifestyle and health practices, activity and rest patterns, environmental toxin exposure, family and social history, and support resources. These data could reveal risk factors for complications.
- ◐ Hormones levels reveal an increase from pre-pregnancy state: hCG, progesterone, estrogen, human placental lactogen, and prostaglandins are increased to maintain pregnancy and prompt alterations in body to prepare for labor and delivery.
- ◐ Genetic testing, particularly if the mother or the father is 35 years old or older.
- ◐ Blood typing and Rh factor testing to determine possible incompatibility between maternal and fetal blood, resulting in destruction of fetal blood cells (erythroblastosis fetalis).
- ◐ Ultrasound with the use of high frequency sound waves to produce a three-dimensional image of internal body structures and tissues. A conducting transducer is used to direct the waves over the abdomen or vaginally toward internal structures. Ultrasound can be done by external abdominal or internal transvaginal approach.
- ◐ Ultrasound is useful to determine several aspects of the pregnancy, including gestational age, fetal growth and viability, maternal pelvic proportions, and placental placement and attachment.

Nurse Alert **To prepare a woman for abdominal ultrasound:**

- • **One to two quarts of fluid should be consumed to fill the bladder.**
- • **Position the woman supine with back supports.**
- • **Warm the conducting gel, if possible, but inform the woman that the gel will be placed on her abdomen and may be cool initially.**

Nurse Alert **To prepare a woman for transvaginal ultrasound:**

- • **Position the woman in a lithotomy position and explain that the probe will be lubricated and inserted into the vagina and that pressure will be felt.**
- • **Explain that the probe will be repositioned as needed to promote visualization of structures.**
- ◐ **Reassure the woman that no harm will come to fetus from the probe or ultrasound waves.**

◑ In gestational trophoblastic disease, after mole evacuation is performed through suction curettage, hCG levels are monitored regularly, and ultrasounds and pelvic exams are performed on a regular basis to determine the presence of a malignancy (choriocarcinoma).

◢6◣ TREATMENTS

◑ Nutritious diet with adequate calories and recommended dietary allowances adjusted as dietary reference intakes (DRI) for pregnant females based on age.

◑ Prenatal vitamins are prescribed to ensure provision of adequate nutrients to the fetus without depriving the mother.

◑ Limited or no over-the-counter medications without clearance from a health-care provider to avoid possible teratogenic medications (which are particularly dangerous in the first and second trimesters).

◑ Complementary and alternative medicine (CAM), including massage, yoga, acupuncture, biofeedback, herbal or other homeopathic medicine, chiropractic treatments, or therapeutic touch may be offered as options to ease the discomforts of pregnancy and promote a sense of well-being.

◑ Treatment for gestational trophoblastic disease involves dilation and curettage (D&C) to remove all products of conception. Postoperative care is provided including monitoring for infection or hemorrhage.

◑ In gestational trophoblastic disease, if high hCG levels and enlarging uterus are noted, and choriocarcinoma is diagnosed, chemotherapy may be administered.

    • If the woman is Rh negative, immune globulin (RhoGAM) is administered to decrease antibody buildup.

◢6◣ NURSING INTERVENTIONS

◑ At the initial contact with the pregnant woman the nurse should explain the process of prenatal visits, including the pelvic exams and blood tests.

Nurse Alert **Consider cultural norms related to pregnancy and childbirth. Accommodate cultural variations if no harm to the mother or fetus is likely. Communicate with the head of household in addition to the client if culturally appropriate to facilitate informed decision making and compliance with care.**

- Provide teaching on fetal development and related changes. Provide nutrition education and assist the mother in incorporating needed nutritional intake into the family diet.
- Encourage daily intake of prescribed prenatal vitamins and iron. Provide strategies to help the mother overcome the side-effects of iron that can cause discomfort, i.e., constipation (encourage fruit and vegetables for fiber).
- Educate the mother and family on the progression of the pregnancy, i.e., fetal development, and the importance of regular prenatal checkups, and changes that will occur in her body as the pregnancy progresses. Discuss strategies to promote comfort:
  a. Supportive bra as breast heaviness increases.
  b. Increased rest for fatigue.
  c. Increase daily fluids and decrease evening intake to minimize nocturia.
  d. Lie on side to reduce pressure of fetus on bladder and major blood vessels.
- Instruct the woman and family regarding abnormal symptoms that might indicate problems in the pregnancy and when to seek medical attention.
- Encourage the expectant mother and father to talk with a caregiver and each other about the pregnancy and to expect that doubts and fears may emerge as they move through the pregnancy (particularly with the first child). Explain that emotional fluctuations are expected and that talking may help in dealing with concerns.
- Discuss preparation for childbirth and provide information about childbirth classes.
- With gestational trophoblastic disease the nurse should:
  a. Assess for risk factors or signs and symptoms: Note rapid increased fundal height measurements, vaginal bleeding, severe hyperemesis, high blood pressure, and edema.
  b. Instruct the client to report and collect specimens of any tissue passed from the vagina for a health-care provider to examine.
  c. Stress the importance of contraception to avoid pregnancy for at least 6 months to allow monitoring for increasing hCG that could indicate malignancy. Instruct the client on the importance of follow-up visits and testing.
  d. Support the client and family in emotional crises related to feelings of loss of a child. Refrain from judgment and do not minimize the client's sense of loss of a child. Explain as often as needed that the mass was not a living fetus, but support their grief.

ROUTINE CHECKUP 1

1. The nurse notes that a woman's fundal measurement is twice as large as expected at the third prenatal visit. The hCG level is high. Which symptom would be most important as an additional sign that the woman might have gestational trophoblastic disease?
   a. Report of increased fetal activity over the past weeks
   b. Report of extreme nausea and vomiting
   c. Swollen breasts with dark nipples and areola
   d. Nosebleeds and nasal stuffiness

Answer:

2. What should the nurse do if a pregnant woman reports urinary frequency that makes it difficult for her to sleep at night?
   a. Instruct the woman to take a mild diuretic in the mornings to reduce fluid.
   b. Encourage the woman to eat watermelon or lemon water prior to going to bed.
   c. Suggest that the woman drink fluids during the day and limit fluid intake at night.
   d. Recommend that the woman limit water intake to three glasses per day.

Answer:

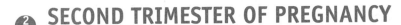

SECOND TRIMESTER OF PREGNANCY

The second trimester involves the period of fetal development from weeks 14 through 24 or 25. Colostrum may be expressed from the breasts beginning in the second trimester. Dizziness and light-headedness might be noted at the beginning of the second trimester because of progesterone and relaxation of the vessels with pooling of blood in the lower extremities (aggravated by pressure from the fetus and with prolonged standing). Additional changes that may occur include the following:

- The woman may gain 1 pound per week for the rest of the pregnancy.
- More energy is noted than in the first trimester.
- Increased vaginal secretions may be noted.

 Nurse Alert **If complaint of itching or unpleasant odor is reported, an infection may be present.**

- Decreased urinary frequency is noted when the uterus lifts out of the pelvic area during the second trimester.
- Increased abdominal size is noted due to the growing fetus, amniotic sac, and uterine size; itching may be noted due to the stretching of skin.
- Skin changes such as striae gravidarum, chloasma, linea nigra, and acne may occur.
- Fetal movement is noted by the woman, with an increased sense that she is truly pregnant.
- Late in the second trimester nosebleeds and nasal stuffiness may occur, as well as straie.
- Many tests that were more dangerous to the fetus earlier can be performed at this point.

5 TEST RESULTS

Doppler blood flow (umbilical velocimetry) may be done to measure the speed of red blood cell flow to detect perfusion problems in the placenta during the second and third trimesters. The peak velocity of the waves, the systolic (S) measure, and the lowest wave point diastolic (D) are noted and the S/D ratio is measured. Normal ratio by 26 weeks gestation is 2.6, and by the end of the pregnancy term it is less than 3. A reading above 3 is abnormal. An abnormal Doppler flow study in addition to low amniotic fluid levels may indicate a risk for the infant being small for its gestational age, having respiratory distress, and having other poor-nutrition-related problems. Doppler studies are done as early as the 16th week and are repeated regularly for high-risk pregnancies.

Amniocentesis is the aspiration of amniotic fluid to assess for fetal abnormalities (such as a genetic condition) or fetal lung maturity. An ultrasound is used to locate the fetus; then a needle is inserted into the uterus to aspirate fluid.

Nurse Alert **Care during and after the procedure includes monitoring vital signs and watching for signs of maternal hypotension or excess venous return, as well as monitoring fetal heart tones for signs of distress (continue monitoring closely for the first 30–60 hours after the procedure). Instruct the woman to monitor and record fetal movement and to report lack of movement immediately; in addition, the woman should note and report any onset of contractions, vaginal drainage, fever, or chills.**

The quadruple screen is a less invasive test for genetic abnormalities such as Down syndrome (trisomy 21), neural tube defects (NTDs), or trisomy 18.

The test assesses the serum levels of substances that may indicate adequate growth and lung development—α-fetoprotein (AFP), human chorionic gonadotropin (hCG), unconjugated estriol (UE3), and diameric inhibin-A. An amniocentesis is needed for definitive diagnosis of the conditions.

Fetal lung maturity: Phospholipids that compose surfactant that lines the alveoli of the lungs, such as lecithin/sphingomyelin (L/S) at a ratio of 2:1, and the presence of phosphatidylglycerol (PG) with associated lamellar body counts (LBCs) of over 32,000 indicate that lung maturity is present.

Chorionic villus sampling (CVS): A sample obtained transabdominally or transcervically from the developing placenta can be used to detect genetic anomalies. This procedure can be done as early as the 10th week of gestation and provides an earlier diagnosis than amniocentesis but carries a higher risk for fetal injury or mortality. Possible complications include ruptured membranes, amniotic fluid leakage, bleeding, infection, and Rh alloimmunization. Due to the early timing of the test, NTDs cannot be detected with this procedure.

A **biophysical profile (BPP)** of the fetus is performed with ultrasound visualization of the fetus combined with a reactive nonstress test to note fetal activity and status. A rating of 2 is a passing score:

- Fetal breathing (one or more episodes of 30-second duration in 30 minutes = 2; less or absent breathing = 0).
- Fetal movement of limbs and body (a minimum of 3 body extensions with return to flexion in 30 minutes = 2; fewer or no movements = 0).
- Fetal tone (at least one episode of limb extension with return flexion = 2; slow or no movement, or absence of flexion = 0).
- Volume of amniotic fluid surrounding fetus: Amniotic fluid index (AFI) is obtained by measuring fluid in the deepest vertical pocket in the 4 quadrants of the uterine area (a minimum of 1 pocket with 2 cm of fluid and AFI >5 cm = 2; less fluid or AFI <5 cm = 0).
- Reactive fetal heart rate with activity (reactive nonstress test [NST]): More than 2 accelerations of >15 beats/min for 15 seconds in 20–40 minutes = 2; 0–1 acceleration in 20–40 minutes = 0.

Treatment

If NST is nonreactive, a diagnostic ultrasound, contraction stress test (CST), and BPP may be ordered. If the fetus is viable, immediate delivery is performed.

WHAT WENT WRONG?

A major complication that can occur early in pregnancy is **incompetent cervix**—the dilation of the cervix without uterine contractions. In this situation the cervix is unable to contain the fetus and opens with the weight of the growing fetus, expelling the fetus and other products of conception. This occurs around 20 weeks of gestation.

Signs and Symptoms

Incompetent cervix may manifest with vaginal drainage or bleeding (possibly a gush of fluids as membranes rupture), pelvic pressure, and contractions and expulsion of the fetus and products of conception.

Test Results

- Ultrasound may reveal a short cervix (less than 20 mm) indicating decreased competence.

Treatments

- In incompetent cervix, if found prior to fetal expulsion, a cervical cerclage—a surgical reinforcement—may be performed to prevent premature dilation. The cerclage remains in place until week 37 of gestation. Activity restrictions or bed rest may be ordered.
- Treatment for incompetent cervix with partial expulsion of the fetus involves a D&C to remove all products of conception—postoperative care is provided including monitoring for infection or hemorrhage.

NURSING INTERVENTIONS

1. Monitor vital signs.
2. In case of incompetent cervix, the nurse should:
    a. Observe for signs of incompetent cervix such as vaginal drainage or bleeding, and reports of pressure with or without contraction.
    b. Encourage hobbies or other distractions to promote compliance with activity restrictions and bed rest, if ordered.
3. Instruct the client and family regarding activity restrictions, including refraining from sexual intercourse, standing for long periods, or heavy lifting.
4. Avoid dehydration, which may stimulate contractions, by promoting regular fluid intake.
5. Instruct the client regarding signs of preterm labor—strong contractions less than 5 minutes apart, rupture of membranes, or perineal pressure with desire to push—and infection.
6. Arrange for a home health nurse and instruct the client in the use of a home uterine activity monitor, if ordered.
7. Instruct the client on the importance of follow-up visits and care.
8. Support the client and family in the emotional crisis related to the loss of a child. Refer for grief counseling, if indicated.

ROUTINE CHECKUP 2

1. What symptoms are common in the second trimester of pregnancy?
   a. Diarrhea
   b. Decreased appetite
   c. Urinary urgency and frequency
   d. Abdominal itching

Answer:

2. What change in the second trimester may have the greatest impact on the woman's psychological adjustment to the pregnancy?
   a. The increased skin sensitivity causes the woman to bond more with the fetus.
   b. The woman can feel the fetal form on her abdomen, making the infant more real.
   c. The extra burst of energy the woman experiences makes it easier to think about the newborn's birth and joining the family.
   d. The first experience of fetal movement makes it clearer that the pregnancy and the fetus are truly present.

Answer:

THIRD TRIMESTER OF PREGNANCY

The third trimester begins after the 24th week and proceeds until delivery of the newborn. Blood pressure stabilizes and dizziness peaks around week 32, then resolves. The problems of the second trimester related to the pressure of the growing fetus; hormone changes, particularly related to back pain; vascular pressures; and gastrointestinal changes are intensified during the final trimester.

- Thoracic breathing becomes more common than abdominal breathing and dyspnea may be noted as the pregnancy progresses and the fundus reaches the xiphoid process.
- As the enlarging fetus exerts pressure against the diaphragm, the chest cavity may enlarge, with progesterone causing relaxation of joints and ligaments. The chest cavity width will increase as the fetal enlargement causes the cavity height to decrease, thus maintaining the cavity capacity and breathing efficiency.
- Indigestion/heartburn may be noted, as well as flatulence and constipation.
- Dependent edema (swollen ankles) and lower extremity, vulva, and rectal varicose veins may develop as the enlarged uterus presses on the femoral veins.

- Swelling and vascular dilation of the lower extremities places the pregnant woman at risk for thrombophlebitis (blood clots).
- Urinary frequency returns as the enlarging uterus presses on the bladder.
- Breasts are enlarged and tender.
- Hemorrhoids may develop.
- The woman's skeletal frame must adjust to the increased weight, and a waddling walk may be noted later in pregnancy as the pelvic joints relax to prepare for delivery. Lordosis may be noted as the woman tries to adjust to the weight of her stomach and breasts.
- Increasing backache is noted as the pregnancy progresses.
- Braxton-Hicks contractions are noted and may intensify in preparation for true labor.

5 TEST RESULTS

The **nonstress test (NST)** is the most commonly used test to evaluate the status of the fetus by measuring fetal heart rate (FHR) during fetal movement. An external transducer is applied to the maternal abdomen to monitor contractions, and a Doppler is used to monitor FHR. When the mother senses fetal movement, a tracing of the FHR is marked to allow analysis. Acoustics or vibration and sound may be used to stimulate movement. This test is most commonly performed in the third trimester. An NST is considered *reactive* if, during fetal activity, two or more times during a 20-minute period the FHR accelerates for at least 15 seconds to a rate of 15 beats per minute. An NST is considered *nonreactive* if the FHR does not accelerate sufficiently with movement or there is no fetal movement in 40 minutes. Further assessment using a contraction stress test (CST) or a BPP should be done.

A **contraction stress test (CST)** is used to determine the flow of oxygenated blood through the placenta during a stimulated or induced contraction. The flow is usually decreased slightly with contractions and normally the fetus adapts and tolerates the decrease. If oxygen reserves are limited, fetal hypoxia and myocardial depression with decreased FHR occurs, indicating that the fetus cannot tolerate the stress of uterine contractions. A baseline of FHR and fetal movement and contractions should be obtained for a 10- to 20-minute period. Then the woman is instructed to brush across her nipples or roll her breast nipples between her finger and thumb (or a mechanical stimulator may be applied) to provide stimulation until a contraction is initiated. If oxytocin is used to induce contractions, monitor closely. A *negative* CST is noted if no late deceleration is noted with 3 contractions of 40 or more seconds in a 10-minute period. A *positive* test shows late decelerations with over half of the contractions, indicating that the fetus is unable to tolerate the stress and as labor progresses fetal distress would develop. If the test results are suspicious with less than 50% of the contractions causing late decelerations, or hyperstimulation occurs with longer (>90 seconds) or more frequent contractions (every 2 minutes) that result in late decelerations, the finding is termed *equivocal* and further testing is needed. An *unsatisfactory* finding results if tracing of FHR is poor or the contractions never reach 3 in 10 minutes with 40-second or longer duration.

Nurse Alert **Caution the mother to stop when contraction is sensed and to rest for periods between testing to prevent uterine hyperstimulation.**

Nurse Alert **CST is contraindicated in placenta previa, abruption placentae, vaginal bleeding of unknown origin, premature rupture of the membranes, incompetent cervix with cerclage intact, abnormal maternal reproductive organs, previous cesarean with vertical incision of the fundus, or history of preterm labor or multiple gestation birth. Review the woman's history carefully.**

WHAT WENT WRONG?

Preterm labor, placenta previa, and abruption placenta may occur late in the second trimester or in the third trimester (see details in Chap. 9).

Signs and Symptoms

- ◗ Vaginal discharge with pink tinge, regular uterine contractions, and cervical dilation and effacement prior to the 36th week of gestation indicates premature labor.
- ◗ Vaginal bleeding that is painless as the cervix dilates (placenta previs) or accompanied by sharp abdominal pain and a rigid uterus (abruption placenta) are signs of major complications.

Test Results

- ◗ Ultrasound indicates the location of the placenta or short cervix in preterm labor.
- ◗ Fetal fibronectin (fFN) via cervical swab may indicate preterm labor.

TREATMENTS

- ◗ Cerclage is removed after week 37 for women with incompetent cervix.
- ◗ Maalox or Mylanta may be permitted to relieve indigestion; sodium bicarbonate is prohibited.
- ◗ See later chapter for detailed care of other complications.

NURSING INTERVENTIONS

- ◐ Encourage the woman to sit with her feet elevated as much as possible.
- ◐ Instruct the woman to rise slowly to minimize dizziness and risk of fall, when noted.
- ◐ Encourage the use of support hose to assist with lower extremity circulation problems.
- ◐ A cool vaporizer may help with respiratory discomfort; the use of petroleum jelly may relieve nosebleeds.
- ◐ Encourage the use of a well-fitting and supportive bra.
- ◐ Skin changes will resolve after pregnancy (except striae); cream may relieve itching and some brands may reduce stretch marks. A gentle soap could remove excess oils and reduce acne.
- ◐ Increased fiber intake, fluid intake, and regular exercise can decrease constipation.
- ◐ Small, frequent meals; avoiding fatty foods; and avoiding lying down after eating may relieve indigestion.
- ◐ Instruct the woman to eat watermelon or drink lemon water (2 tbsp/ glass) to encourage diuresis and reduce swelling.
- ◐ Pelvic tilt exercises may strengthen back and abdominal muscles and reduce back pain; low-heeled shoes are encouraged.
- ◐ Instruct the woman to lie on her side when sleeping to minimize pressure on major vessels and improve fetal circulation.
- ◐ Address concerns of the woman and family regarding labor and delivery; encourage preparation classes.
- ◐ Educate the woman and family on postdelivery needs and on caring for a newborn.

✔ ROUTINE CHECKUP 3

1. Why might a woman in the third trimester of pregnancy experience greater urinary frequency than noted in the second trimester?

Answer:

---

2. What finding would be unusual for a woman in her third trimester of pregnancy?
   a. Sleeplessness
   b. Braxton-Hicks contractions
   c. Painful backache
   d. Vaginal bleeding

Answer:

CONCLUSION

The body of the pregnant female undergoes a significant number of changes over the duration of the pregnancy. Some changes and complications are more common during specific pregnancy periods. These periods, trimesters, are divided into approximately 12-week intervals. This chapter reviewed the maternal changes experienced as the pregnancy proceeds from the first to the third trimester and related nursing care needed to support a healthy pregnancy and address complications that may occur:

First trimester: Conception to the 12th or 13th week of gestation:
◐ The signs of pregnancy can be:
- Presumptive signs, which include subjective or objective signs:
  ◦ Amenorrhea
  ◦ Nausea and vomiting
  ◦ Fatigue
  ◦ Urinary frequency
  ◦ Quickening
  ◦ Uterine enlargement
  ◦ Linea nigra
  ◦ Cholasma
  ◦ Striae gravidarum
  ◦ Breast changes
  ◦ Darkened areola
- Probable signs, which include changes seen during the assessment that lead to the suspicion of pregnancy:
  ◦ Goodell's sign: Softening of the cervix
  ◦ Hegar's sign: Softening and increased flexibility of the lower uterus
  ◦ Chadwick's sign
  ◦ Ballottement
  ◦ Positive pregnancy test: Detected hCG
  ◦ Palpable fetal outline
  ◦ Braxton-Hicks contractions
  ◦ Cervical changes
  ◦ Abdominal enlargement

Two methods may be used to determine the delivery date:
◐ Nagele's rule: Take the first day of the last menstrual cycle, subtract 3 months, and add 7 days and 1 year.
◐ McDonald's method: Gestational age is equal to the fundal height.

Physiologic changes over the three trimesters may include the following:
◐ Menstrual cycle stops.
◐ Nausea and vomiting in early pregnancy.
◐ Integumentary/skin changes, such as striae and cholasma.

- Nasal stuffiness and nosebleeds.
- Increased blood volume and heart rate.
- Pseudoanemia.
- Increased respiratory workload.
- Breast changes (engorgement and hyperpigmentation).
- Reflux, heartburn, and constipation.
- Urinary frequency.
- Diminished hearing.

Tests that may be used in pregnancy include the following:

- Hormone levels
- Ultrasound
- Genetic testing
- Blood typing (including Rh factor)
- Doppler blood flow
- Amniocentesis
- Quadruple screen
- Lecithin/sphingomyelin (L/S) ratio of 2:1, and phosphatidylglycerol (PG) with associated lamellar body counts (LBCs) to determine fetal lung maturity
- Chorionic villus sampling (CVS)
- Biophysical profile (BPP)
- Nonstress test (NST)
- Contraction stress test (CST)

Complications that may occur prior to or in the early stage of pregnancy include the following:

First trimester

- Gestational trophoblastic disease
- Spontaneous abortion
- Ectopic pregnancy
- Hyperemesis gravidarum (HEG)

Second trimester

- Incompetent **cervix**

Third trimester

- Preterm labor
- Placenta previa
- Abruption placenta

Monitoring for the expected changes of pregnancy assists the nurse in validating that the pregnancy is progressing well since many changes are associated with fetal growth. Assessing for signs of complications of pregnancy promotes early interventions that might stop the complication from progressing and decrease the negative impact on mother and fetus.

? FINAL CHECKUP

1. **The patient history records that a woman is gravida 3 para 2, which indicates that the woman has had which of the following?**
   a. Two pregnancies with three births after the fetus was at 20 weeks gestation or older.
   b. Two pregnancies with three live births with the fetus at 20 weeks gestation or older.
   c. Three pregnancies with two births after the fetus was at 20 weeks gestation or older.
   d. Three pregnancies with two abortions with the fetus at 20 weeks gestation or older.

2. **A woman has been told she is not pregnant but has gestational trophoblastic disease. She asks the nurse, "Did my baby die?" What would be the best response by the nurse?**
   a. "There was no baby; you had a growth like a cancer tumor."
   b. "The cells that might have become a baby never developed."
   c. "Yes, your baby died because of the trophoblastic disease."
   d. "You should not worry; you can try to get pregnant again."

3. **Which of the following women would the nurse watch most carefully for signs of gestational trophoblastic disease?**
   a. Miss Kelly, age 20, who is having her first baby
   b. Mrs. Deeds, age 32, who is having her third baby
   c. Mrs. Beal, age 37, who is having her second child
   d. Miss Davies, age 28, who is having her fourth child

4. **Miss Kelly, age 20, who is having her first child, reports to the clinic with complaints of "vomiting every morning but then being really hungry." The nurse could provide which of the following explanations to Miss Kelly?**
   a. The vomiting is a sign that something might be wrong and it should be reported to the doctor.
   b. The vomiting is a nervous reaction to being pregnant; it will subside after you accept the pregnancy.
   c. The increased levels of hCG in response to the pregnancy causes nausea and vomiting.
   d. Tell Miss Kelly she is experiencing the nausea and vomiting because this is her first pregnancy.

5. **A woman reports to the emergency room with concerns that her pregnancy "is not going well" because the baby is not moving. She is at 26 weeks gestation. Which of the following tests is most likely to be ordered for assessment of the fetus to address the woman's concerns?**
   a. Biophysical profile and reactive nonstress test
   b. Chorionic villus sampling
   c. Fetal lung maturity
   d. The quadruple screen and chorionic villus sampling

6. **Monica Bailey, age 30, is at 29 weeks gestation and undergoes a nonstress test. Which of the following statements is true about diagnostic testing in pregnancy?**
   a. If the nonstress test is reactive, a diagnostic ultrasound and BPP may be ordered.
   b. If the nonstress test is reactive, the fetus that is at viable age is delivered immediately.
   c. If the nonstress test is nonreactive, a contraction stress test and BPP may be ordered.
   d. If the nonstress test is nonreactive, the pregnancy is terminated because the fetus is not viable.

7. **Which of the following women would be most likely to undergo chorionic villus sampling?**
   a. Penny Marshall, age 19, first pregnancy
   b. Bonnie Veal, age 29, first pregnancy
   c. Sara Eaton, age 34, first pregnancy
   d. Patricia Dennis, age 38, first pregnancy

8. **A woman in her second trimester of pregnancy reports to the emergency room with concerns that she is "losing this baby just like she did a year ago." The ultrasound reveals a cervix that is less than 20 mm. Which of the following conditions and treatments should the nurse prepare the woman for?**
   a. Incompetent cervix, which will be treated with delivery of the fetus
   b. Cervical effacement, which will be treated with topical oxytocin
   c. Incompetent cervix, which will be treated with cervical cerclage
   d. Cervical effacement, which will be treated with delivery of the fetus

9. **A woman in her third trimester of pregnancy indicates that she has increased pressure on her bladder but less pressure on her lungs than she did a few weeks ago. The nurse would respond in which of the following ways?**
   a. Instruct the woman to sit down and prepare for strict bed rest because the baby has begun a premature descent for birth that must be stopped or premature birth will follow.
   b. Inform the woman that as the baby moves into position for delivery the weight shifts downward, relieving pressure on the lungs but causing pressure on the bladder.
   c. Inform the primary-care provider that the woman is experiencing a major complication and prepare for immediate delivery.
   d. Assess breath sounds and obtain a urine specimen to determine if the pulmonary nerves have been paralyzed and a urinary tract infection is present.

10. **During the third trimester, what measures may be used to address discomforts of pregnancy?**
    a. Decreased dietary fiber will reduce the flatulence that often occurs in late pregnancy.
    b. Weight-lifting exercises may strengthen back and abdominal muscles.
    c. Lie on back when sleeping to reduce renal blood flow and urinary frequency.
    d. Lemon water may be ingested to stimulate diuresis to reduce swelling.

ANSWERS

Routine Checkup 1
1. b
2. c

Routine Checkup 2
1. d
2. d

Routine Checkup 3
1. The fundus begins to drop in the pelvis, placing weight on the bladder.
2. d

Final Checkup

1. c	2. b	3. c	4. c
5. a	6. c	7. d	8. c
9. b	10. d		

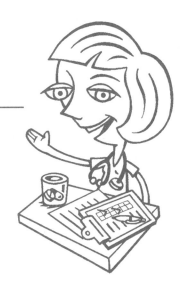

CHAPTER 7

Fetal Development

Objective

At the end of this chapter, the student will be able to:

1 Discuss the progression of the fertilized egg from conception to birth.

2 Review the changes that occur during each 2–4 week span during pregnancy.

3 Evaluate assessments and diagnostic findings associated with fetal development.

4 Discuss nursing interventions that promote a healthy pregnancy and birth.

5 Identify conditions and circumstances that can interfere with fetal development.

6 Discuss the treatment and nursing interventions needed to support the newborn, parents, and families when altered fetal development occurs.

KEY TERMS

Cephalocaudal	Polydactyly
Dizygotic	Postconception age
Ductus arteriosus	Preembryonic stage
Embryonic stage	Quickening
Fetal stage	Shoulder dystocia
Foramen ovale	Somites
Lanugo	Syndactyly
Macrosomic	Teratogens
Monozygotic	Vernix caseosa
Omphalocele	

OVERVIEW

After conception occurs, the zygote progresses to an embryo and then becomes a fetus. Generally, the growth period from fertilization to birth is considered to be 2 weeks less than the gestational age or length of pregnancy calculated from the onset of the most recent regular menstrual period to the time of birth, 280 days or 40 weeks duration. The **postconception age** is calculated to be about 266 days or 91/2 months. At each stage of fetal development, distinct physical changes occur and can be noted upon ultrasound examination. The fetus is vulnerable to many factors that can impair or alter development, particularly in the early stages of development. Assessment at each stage of fetal development promotes early detection of problems that may arise. Nursing care is directed at promotion of healthy fetal development and prevention or reduction of dangerous maternal behaviors and fetal exposures that could result in fetal morbidity or mortality.

   As stated in chapter 4, the fertilized egg is called a zygote.

   ❶ The first two weeks after conception are called the germinal period, during which the cells continue to duplicate and the zygote moves through the fallopian tubes to the uterus. The first 2 weeks of development are considered the **preembryonic stage**.

   ❶ The **embryonic stage** begins at day 15 and proceeds through week 8 or about 56 days.

   ❶ The final stage is the **fetal stage**, which continues from the beginning of week 9 through birth (Fig. 7.1).

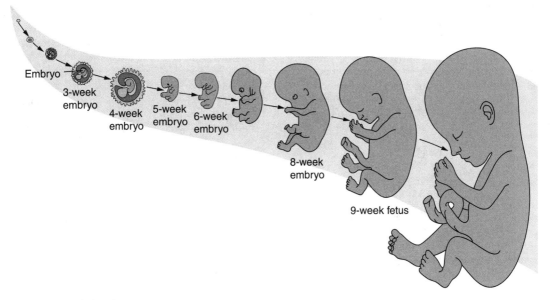

Figure 7.1 • Fetal development.

◉ During the embryonic and fetal stages, the head and back are flexed and length is measured from the top of the head (crown-C) to the bottom of the hips (rump-R).

◉ In the fetal stage, as extremities grow longer, the measurement from crown to heel (C-H) is also taken.

👉 The major fetal development (in postconception weeks) that occurs during the embryonic and fetal stages include the following (**Table 7.1**)

THE EMBRYONIC STAGE

From approximately day 10 to day 14 after conception and during the embryonic stage the germ cell layers, the ectoderm, mesoderm, and endoderm are formed as membranes from which tissues, organs, and organ systems grow. At this stage the embryo is most vulnerable to cell and tissue damage from **teratogens** (agents that can cause damage to a developing fetus such as drugs, infections, or radiation). The ectoderm forms a cylinder-shaped tube that will form the brain and spinal cord. The gastrointestinal (GI) tract develops from the endoderm and forms another cylinder that attaches to the yolk sac. A tube-shaped heart forms outside the body initially, and by the end of the 7th week blood cells will circulate through major blood vessels. Red blood

TABLE 7.1 • Fetal Development in Postconception Weeks					
Age in Wks	Length and Weight	Body and Organ Formation	Neurologic/ Sensory	Cardiovascular and Respiratory	Gastrointestinal/ Endocrine	Genital/ Urinary
2–3	The fetal length crown to rump (C-R) is 2 mm	Optic cup and lens, eye pigment/ auditory cavities form	Neural tube forms from closure of the mid-back groove	Tubular heart begins to form, primitive blood cell circulation begins Nasal cavities form	Liver begins function Thyroid tissue noted	Kidney formation begins
4	Length (C-R) is 4–6 mm Weight 0.4 g	Fetal body is flexed in a C-shaped position Limb (arm/leg) buds noted	Neural tube closes to form brain and spinal cord	A fetal heartbeat is present	Oral cavity, jaws esophagus/ trachea stomach, intestine, ducts of pancreas and liver form	
5	Length (C-R) is 8 mm	Muscles develop with innervation	Brain begins to differentiate and cranial nerves are noted	Atria of the heart divide		
6	Length (C-R) is 12 mm	Bones begin skeletal form Skull/jaw ossification, muscle mass develops	Ear structures form: external, middle, and internal	Heart chambers present, blood cell types can be identified. Trachea bronchi and lung buds	Oral and nasal pits and upper lip form. Liver forms blood cells	Embryonic sex glands appear
7	Length (C-R) is 18 mm		Optic nerve Eyelids form Lens thickens	Fetal heart beat detected, true blood circulation Diaphragm separates the thoracic and abdominal cavities	Tongue separates palate folds Stomach form completed	Bladder and urethra separate from rectum Sex glands differ-entiate to ovaries or testes

TABLE 7.1 • Fetal Development in Postconception Weeks (*Continued*)						
Age in Wks	Length and Weight	Body and Organ Formation	Neurologic/ Sensory	Cardiovascular and Respiratory	Gastrointestinal/ Endocrine	Genital/ Urinary
8	Length (C-R) is 2.5–3 cm Weight 2 g	Digits form Skeleton ossification of bone cartilage Musculature development Movement possible		Fetal heart rate can usually be heard by Doppler		
10	Length (C-H) is 5–6 cm Weight 14 g	Finger and toe nails begin to grow		Brain divisions in place, neurons at end of spinal cord	Lips separate from jaw, palate folds fuse, intestines become enclosed in abdomen Islets of Langerhans form	Bladder sac developed Male testos-terone and physical charac-teristics
12	Length 8 cm (C-R) C-H = 11.5 cm Weight 45 g	Skin thin and pink Bones more evident with full skeletal ossification Involuntary visceral muscles	Lymphoid tissue appears in thymus gland	Lungs have clear shape and form	Palate is formed Gut muscles Bile secretion Liver produces blood cells Thyroid, pancreas secrete hormones	Renal function begins with urine formation by kidneys Gender of the fetus can usually be deter-mined by ultra-sound

(*Continued*)

TABLE 7.1 • Fetal Development in Postconception Weeks *(Continued)*						
Age in Wks	Length and Weight	Body and Organ Formation	Neurologic/ Sensory	Cardiovascular and Respiratory	Gastrointestinal/ Endocrine	Genital/ Urinary
16	Length 13.5 cm (C-R) C-H = 15 cm Weight 200 g	Skin, **lanugo** (fine soft hair) over the body, sweat glands Hair on scalp Teeth form hard tissue Eyes, ears, nose formed	Sensory organs can be distinguished	Heart muscle is fully formed Fetal heart tone audible with fetoscope (at 16–20 wks) Blood vessels visible	Hard and soft palate evident Gastric and intestinal glands Meconium forms in intestines	Kidneys shaped Gender can be determined
20	Length 19 cm (C-R) C-H = 25 cm Weight 435 g 6% body fat	Lanugo on total body, brown fat forms, waxy skin coating (**vernix caseosa**) develops Lower limbs become proportional Bone marrow function increases, iron is stored Teeth form hard tissue that will be canines and molars	Fetal brain development continues Spinal cord myelination starts Fetal (IgG) antibodies noted	Heartbeat can be auscultated with the fetoscope Respiratory movement is initiated	Fetus sucks and swallows Peristaltic activity begins	
24	Length 23 cm (C-R) C-H = 28 cm Weight 780 g	Skin red in color and wrinkled, vernix caseosa Teeth form hard tissue that will be second molars	Brain appears like a mature brain Fetal IgG reaches maternal levels	Respiratory movement regular (24–40 wks), nostrils open, alveoli produce surfactant, gas exchange capable		

TABLE 7.1 • Fetal Development in Postconception Weeks (*Continued*)						
Age in Wks	Length and Weight	Body and Organ Formation	Neurologic/ Sensory	Cardiovascular and Respiratory	Gastrointestinal/ Endocrine	Genital/ Urinary
28	Length 27 cm (C-R) C-H = 35 cm Weight 1200– 1250 g	Adipose tissue accumulates, nails present Eyelids open, eyebrows and eye lashes intact	Nervous system regulation of some body functions begins Weak suck reflex	Respiratory movement present		Testes descend into upper scrotum and inguinal canal
32	Length 31 cm (C-R) C-H = 38– 43 cm Weight 2000 g	Subcutaneous fat building	Many reflexes present Sense of taste in place Awareness of sounds outside maternal body noted			
36	Length 35 cm (C-R) C-H = 42– 48 cm Weight 2500– 2750 g	Pale skin, rounded body Decreased lanugo, hair fuzzy Distal femoral ossification centers noted				
38-40	Length 40 cm (C-R) C-H = 48– 52 cm Weight >3200 g 16% body fat	Smooth skin with pink undertones, vernix in skin folds, lanugo on shoulders and upper back Earlobes firm due to cartilage Nails extend over tips of digits		Ratio of lecithin-sphingomyelin (L/S ratio) near 2:1 by 38 weeks Adequate surfactant		Males: testes in scrotum or at inguinal canal Females: well-developed labia majora, small labia minora

cells are formed by a yolk sac that develops in the first weeks and continues to function until liver function is established. This sac is later incorporated into the umbilical cord.

Around weeks 4 and 5, mesodermal blocks (**somites**) line both sides of the midline of the embryo and provide the foundation to form the vertebrae of the spinal column. The bases for the lower jaw, hyoid bone, and larynx are developed in this stage. By week 5 the brain has 5 distinct areas and 10 cranial nerve pairs can be noted. By week 6 the heart has most of its major aspects and fetal circulation is established, and true blood cells are produced by the liver. By the end of week 7 the foundation for all internal and external body parts is in place. By the end of week 8, all body structures, organs, and systems are in place. The musculoskeletal frame begins to form. The function of these structures will be refined during the remaining months until birth.

THE FETAL STAGE

During the fetal stage, organ forms and functions are refined. Tooth buds form and the face of the fetus is formed and looks human. The fetal heart rate is 120 to 160 beats per minute. Between weeks 12 and 16 the fetus grows rapidly with musculoskeletal tissue development, which enables movement. By week 20 the fetus becomes active and the mother experiences fetal mobility (**quickening**). By 24 weeks the fetus has a proportioned, lean body. Amniotic fluid contains a respiratory marker (lecithin) that can be used to determine lung maturity. The fetus appears to be able to hear and progresses to awareness of the environment outside the maternal body. In week 28 the eyes of the fetus begin to open and close. The brain is formed and a weak suck reflex is present. By week 32 subcutaneous, brown fat insulation is present. The fetus has fingernails and toenails in place. By week 36 and beyond the fetal body shape is round, skin has pink undertones, and fine lanugo is noted on the upper body. Scant vernix caseosa may be present at full term. The immune system is developing and the newborn is protected by antibodies passed from the mother during this vulnerable period.

FETAL CIRCULATION

Fetal circulation is designed to allow blood flow from the mother through the placenta through the fetal body, but bypassing the nonfunctioning fetal lungs as well as the fetal liver. The fetus receives oxygenated blood and nutrients from the mother and sends deoxygenated blood to the mother for gas exchange to remove carbon dioxide and waste. Blood flows from the placenta to the inferior vena cava and right atrium, then most of the blood flows through the **foramen ovale**, an opening between the fetal atria, into the left atrium and then into the left ventricle and is pumped out through the aorta to the body. A small amount of blood flows from the head and upper extremities into the

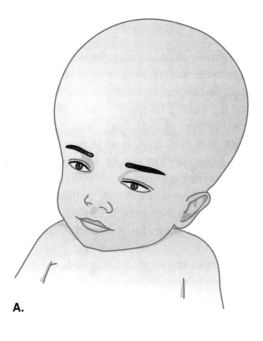

A.

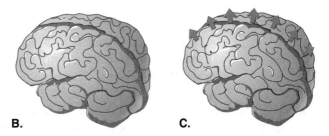

B.   **C.**

Figure 7.2 • A. Enlarged head B. Brain with normal ventricles C. Brain with enlarged ventricles.

right atria and a small amount into the right ventricles. Most blood flows past the lungs and into the aorta and then returns to the placenta through the **ductus arteriosus**, a connection between the pulmonary artery and the aorta that shunts blood past the fetal lungs.

The fetal circulation delivers oxygen to the body in a head-to-toe (**cephalocaudal**) direction, which encourages developmental priority to the brain and heart followed by GI tract and extremities. At birth the flow of fetal circulation is altered when the fetal lungs become functional and blood flow must travel through the lungs for gas exchange. Problems are encountered if fetal heart structures that are designed to shunt blood past the lungs fail to close (see Chap. 12: Newborn Care).

MULTIPLE FETUSES

Multiple fetuses may develop from separate ova/eggs being fertilized by separate spermatozoa (fraternal/**dizygotic**). In this situation two placenta, two chorions, and two amnions form. The fetuses are considered fraternal and do not look the same. Multiple fetuses may also develop from one fertilized ovum (maternal/**monozygotic**). The fetuses share the chorion and placenta, are the same sex, and are identical in appearance. The cellular mass must separate into two or more distinct zygotes for multiple fetuses to develop. If this separation occurs early, individual amnions and chorions will develop. If the separation occurs later the embryos will share the chorion but have separate amnion sacs. If the separation occurs even later after the amnion is formed, a rare occurrence, the fetuses will share the same amnion sac. The development of multiple fetuses is similar to that of a single fetus. Congenital anomalies or defects, secondary to exposure to a teratogen noted in one of the fetuses, are commonly found in all the multiple fetuses in that pregnancy.

DISRUPTION OF FETAL DEVELOPMENT

Rh or ABO incompatibility, as discussed in Chap. 3, can occur when the mother is Rh-negative and the father is Rh-positive. If the fetus is Rh-positive like the father, upon exposure to the baby's blood the mother can develop antibodies that will attack the fetus's blood as a foreign body. The first pregnancy, whether completed to a live birth or ending in an abortion or miscarriage, will sensitize the mother's system and antibodies will be formed, unless the woman was treated with an Rh immune globulin (RhoGAM), which provides passive antibody protection against the Rh antigen and prevents the body from producing its own antibodies. If the mother has been sensitized and has not been treated, the fetus is at risk of having red blood cells destroyed by the mother's antibodies. The fetus may become severely anemic due to red blood cell destruction (hemolysis) and require early delivery (delayed if possible until after 36th or 37th week), or intrauterine transfusions or transfusions immediately after birth. The fetus may also develop ascites, subcutaneous edema, increased heart size, or hydramnios (excess amniotic fluid) and require supportive treatment.

Nursing care is focused on prevention through early assessment for risk and treatment of the woman with each pregnancy. Upon receipt of test results, the nurse should report that the pregnant woman is Rh-negative (indirect Coombs' test is negative, nonsensitized) and fetus is Rh-positive (direct Coombs' test is negative) and follow through with RhoGAM treatment as ordered. Observation should be continued to determine treatment effectiveness and absence of fetal distress due to incompatibility and damage to fetal red blood cells from maternal antibodies.

6 **ABO incompatibility** presents a similar dilemma to that discussed above. Most commonly if the maternal blood type is O (no A or B antigens) and the fetal blood type is A, B, or AB, the fetal antigens are likely to cause the mother to produce antibodies against the fetal blood and hemolysis can occur in the fetus. The anemia is not as severe as with Rh incompatibility and no treatment is available. Additionally, each pregnancy stands alone; thus, no earlier sensitization will impact the current pregnancy. The newborn is monitored upon birth for signs of hyperbilirubinemia which can result from excessive red blood cell death and appropriate treatment is provided.

Teratogens, anything that can interfere with normal fetal development, can cause varied disruptions in fetal body formation. The impact may vary based on when and to what degree the exposure occurred, what tissue was most affected, and fetal genotype, which determines how vulnerable the fetus is to the teratogen. The earlier the exposure to the teratogen, the more disruption occurs to fetal development. If disruption is severe, the fetus does not survive and spontaneous abortion occurs. The most common disruptions include the following:

- Nutritional deficits can cause decreased brain growth and neural tube development (spinal cord disruption), coronary heart disease, diabetes, hypertension, and small or disproportionate fetal body development.
- Maternal hyperthermia can cause central nervous system (CNS) defects or failed neural tube closure.
- Exposure to substance abuse, infection, or a teratogen can result in varied disruptions including mental retardation or body structure malformation depending on the week of exposure, for example:
  - Week 3: Absence of one or more extremities, heart remains outside chest
  - Week 4: Herniation of abdominal structures into umbilical cord (**omphalocele**)
  - Week 5: Cataract, small eyeballs (microphthalmia), facial clefts
  - Week 6: Septal or aortic abnormalities, cleft lip, agnathia (absence of lower jaw)
  - Week 7: Ventricular septal defect, cleft palate, brachycephalism (short head), confused sexual characteristics, pulmonary stenosis
  - Week 8: Persistent atrial septum opening, short fingers or toes

NEURAL TUBE DEFECTS

5 WHAT WENT WRONG?

The neural tube develops into the brain and the spinal cord. A neural tube defect is the failure of the neural tube to close within 28 days after conception in an area of the neural tube or the entire length of the neural tube, resulting in a neurologic disorder in the fetus.

The cause of neural tube defects is unknown; however, there is a link between inadequate intake of folic acid prior to pregnancy and during the first trimester. The most common neural tube defects are:

- Spina bifida occulta: This is the incomplete closure without the spinal cord or meninges protruding. This patient usually doesn't experience neurologic dysfunction, although there might be bladder or bowel disturbances or weakness in the foot.
- Spina bifida cystica: This is the incomplete closure with the spinal cord or meninges protruding in a sac. There are two types of spina bifida cystica. These are:
  - Myelomeningocele: The sac contains the spinal cord, cerebral spinal fluid, and meninges. This patient usually experiences neurologic dysfunction.
  - Meningocele: The sac contains cerebral spinal fluid and the meninges. This patient rarely experiences neurologic dysfunction.
- Anencephaly: Cerebral hemispheres of the brain and the top portion of the skull. The brain stem is intact, enabling the infant to have cardiopulmonary functions; however, the infant is likely to die of respiratory failure a few weeks after birth.
- Encephalocele: Portions of the brain and meninges protrudes in the sac. This patient usually experiences neurologic dysfunction.

SIGNS AND SYMPTOMS

- Spina bifida occulta:
  - Tuft of hair in the lumbar or sacral area
  - Depression in the lumbar or sacral area
  - Hemangioma in the lumbar or sacral area
- Spina bifida cystica meningocele:
  - Presence of sac
- Spina bifida cystica myelomeningocele:
  - Presence of sac
  - Bowel incontinence
  - Bladder incontinence
  - Hydrocephalus
  - Spastic paralysis
  - Club foot
  - Knee contractures
  - Curvature of the spine
  - Arnold-Chiari malformation
- Anencephaly:
  - The top portion of the skull is missing.
- Encephalocele:
  - Mental retardation

- Paralysis
- Hydrocephalus

TEST RESULTS

- Maternal serum tested for α-fetoprotein (MSAFP) serum test: Performed at 15–22 weeks (high levels associated with neural tube defects, anencephaly, omphalocele, or **gastroschisis** (intestines exposed and outside the abdominal wall).
- Aminocentesis: Assess if α-fetoprotein is in amniotic fluid. This test is performed if the α-fetoprotein test is abnormal.
- Ultrasound: Assess if there is a neural tube defect or defect in the ventral wall. This test is performed if the α-fetoprotein test is abnormal.
- Transillumination of the sac: Differentiates between myelomeningocele and meningocele. A meningocele sac does not transilluminate. This test is performed if the sac is present after birth.
- CT scan: Assess the presence of a neural tube defect after birth.
- X-ray: Assess the presence of a neural tube defect after birth.

TREATMENTS

- Surgery within 48 hours of birth to close the opening to decrease the risk of infection and prevent spinal cord damage.
- Insert a shunt to relieve hydrocephalus.

Nurse Alert **Surgery does not reverse the disorder.**

NURSING INTERVENTIONS

- Prenatal:
  - Encourage the mother to take adequate amounts of folic acid during childbearing years.
  - Explain the disorder and treatment following birth.
- After birth:
  - Lay the infant on his or her side to prevent pressure on the sac.
  - Keep the sac covered with a sterile dressing soaked in warmed saline solution to keep the sac moist.
  - Place a strip of plastic below the sac to prevent contamination from urine and stool to prevent infection.
  - Measure head circumference to determine if hydrocephalus develops.
  - Monitor for infection around the sac.
  - Assess for leakage around the sac.
  - Assess bladder and blow function.
  - Assess neurologic signs.
  - Reposition the patient every 2 hours to prevent pressure ulcers and contractures.

- Explain to the family that surgery will be performed to close the opening within 48 hours following birth.
- After surgery:
  - Monitor vital signs.
  - Monitor for signs of infection.
  - Reposition the patient every 2 hours to prevent pressure ulcers from developing.
  - Monitor bowel and bladder function to assess for changes from the preoperative period.
  - Assess neurologic signs.
  - Measure head circumference to determine if hydrocephalus develops.
  - Be prepared to insert a straight urinary catheter if the infant is not urinating adequately.
  - Perform range of motion exercises to maintain muscle tone.

GENETIC ABNORMALITIES

Hereditary conditions can be passed on through the genes of the mother, father, or both. When the ovum and spermatozoa join, on occasion either the egg or sperm may have an extra copy of a chromosome (trisomic) totaling 47 chromosomes. The most common chromosome that is duplicated is number 21. Down syndrome is the most common condition (trisomy 21). The most common consequence of this anomaly is intellectual retardation. Trisomy 13 and 18 may occur, but are both associated with death in the first 3 months of life. Some conditions involve the absence of a chromosome (monosomy), totaling 45. Chromosomal structure anomalies may be found in combination with trisomy conditions. In some cases, after fertilization two different cell lines will develop: one with an abnormal chromosomal number and one with a normal number. This condition should be suspected if symptoms of Down syndrome are noted but intelligence is normal or almost normal. Sex chromosome anomalies can occur if the fetus gets an extra X chromosome (Klinefelter—47, XXY) or female (Turner—45, XO). While individual manifestations of chromosomal anomalies may vary, some common signs and symptoms are noted with the major conditions (**Table 7.2**).

CONGENITAL ANOMALIES

Genetic conditions were discussed in Chapter 4 but will be briefly reviewed here. Some congenital anomalies are inherited conditions that occur as a result of a dominant gene or recessive gene carried by the mother, father, or both. These anomalies could also occur from a sex-linked (X-linked) inheritance. Conditions that occur secondary to inheritance include Huntington's disease, polycystic kidney disease, cystic fibrosis, phenylketonuria (PKU), sickle cell anemia, hemophilia,

TABLE 7.2 • Common Signs and Symptoms of Major Conditions	
Condition	Symptoms
Trisomy 21, 18, 13	Mental retardation, hypotonia, (seizures in trisomy 13); congenital heart disease (see section below for additional data)
Trisomy 18 Trisomy 18, 13 Trisomy 13	Prominent occiput, low set ears, ptosis, **syndactyly** (webbed fingers) Gastrointestinal tract anomalies, malformation of other organs. Microcephaly, malformed ears, cleft lip/palate, **polydactyly** (extra digits)
Turner (XO) females	No intellectual impairment, perceptual difficulties, low hairline, short stature, excessive nevi (skin pigmentation discoloration), wide chest with spaced nipples, no toe nails, fibrous streaked ovaries, underdeveloped secondary sex characteristics, infertility, renal anomalies
Klinefelter (XXY) males	Mild retardation, gynecomastia, lack of male musculature, underdeveloped secondary sex characteristics, infertile/sterile

and Duchenne muscular dystrophy. Some conditions occur secondary to multiple factors combining genes and environment, greater the number of defects the higher the number of factors impacting the fetus. Such conditions include spina bifida, myelomeningocele, or pyloric stenosis. Congenital heart defects will be covered in Chapter 12 with care of the newborn.

 ROUTINE CHECKUP

1. A parent of a Down syndrome child calls saying that she has doubts about the diagnosis because her 2-month-old seems to act like her other child when she was 2 months old. What is the best response?
   a. "Call your health-care provider and ask to have your child retested."
   b. "Your child has Down syndrome according to the child's test results."
   c. "Behavioral differences are not easily noticeable until later in the infant's development."
   d. "Your child has the facial characteristics of a child who has Down syndrome; therefore, your child has the disorder."

Answer:

2. What would the nurse advise a pregnant woman to do to prevent fetal exposure to infection?

Answer:

ALTERATIONS IN FETAL GROWTH

Some pregnancies are identified as high risk because of maternal condition or prenatal exposures that can impact fetal growth. Any condition that could affect maternal nutrition, such as low socioeconomic status, homelessness, or adolescence, or any condition that would disrupt placental delivery of nutrient-rich blood, such as a small placenta or placenta previa, could cause deficits in fetal nutrition. Exposure to environmental factors such as toxins, X-rays, or hyperthermia, or to infections such as toxoplasmosis, other infections, rubella, cytomegalovirus, and herpes simplex virus (TORCH) can increase the risk of fetal growth disturbance. Conditions that impact maternal blood flow would similarly cause a disruption of placental blood flow, for example, maternal heart disease, substance abuse (including tobacco or alcohol use), sickle cell anemia, lupus erythematosis, or phenylketonuria (PKU). Premature newborns (less than 37 weeks) are likely to be small for gestational age (SGA), and postmature newborns (greater than 42 weeks) may be large for gestational age (LGA). Newborns with either designation are at higher risk for complications than newborns that are full term (37–42 weeks) and appropriate for gestational age (AGA). Neonatal risk charting of weeks of gestation and weight in grams has been used to determine the likelihood of morbidity, with premature birth and low weight contributing to a high degree of morbidity and mortality. The evaluation of newborn weight will require consideration of the race of the newborn and standard birth weights for that population.

PRETERM NEWBORN

WHAT WENT WRONG?

A newborn is considered preterm if it is born before completion of the full 37 weeks of gestation. These infants often also have low birth weight (LBW), and occurrence of premature, LBW infants is higher in adolescents and in the African American population. The primary problems with premature LBW infants result from immature systems with decreased function. The stress of birth is a major challenge that some premature infants do not survive. A number of problems challenge premature infants.

SIGNS AND SYMPTOMS, AND TEST RESULTS

 Nurse Alert **When evaluating developmental accomplishments, the newborn should be assessed based on chronological age from expected date of birth from conception, not actual date of birth.**

◗ Respiratory system:
- The premature newborn has low amounts of surfactant, resulting in alveoli that collapse easily and leading to poor gas exchange and decreased oxygenation, hypoxia, and poor activity tolerance due to low oxygen reserves. Respiratory distress syndrome (RDS) can result and requires intensive treatment (see Chap. 12: Newborn Care).
- Increased flow of blood back into the lungs through the ductus arteriosus, which fails to close after birth because oxygen levels and prostaglandin E levels do not increase sufficiently to stimulate vasoconstriction of the ductus arteriosus. A resulting pulmonary congestion, carbon dioxide retention, bounding femoral pulses, and increased respiratory effort are noted. Pulmonary dysfunction can become chronic.
- Apnea of prematurity (cessation of breathing for up to 20 seconds or less than 20 seconds, accompanied by bradycardia, cyanosis, or pallor) may be noted secondary to immature neurologic control of respirations, or obstruction from structural collapse or secretions.

◗ Poor temperature control:
- High body surface for low body weight, which provides high loss of heat with lower heat production resulting in newborn hypothermia.
- Decreased subcutaneous fat, resulting in minimum insulation and increased loss of body heat from blood vessels that are close to the skin surface.
- Thin skin with high permeability, leading to water loss and heat loss.
- Premature newborn posture with less flexion and greater extension of limbs leads to greater exposure of body surface area and greater heat loss.
- The newborn's ability to vasoconstrict blood vessels is decreased, causing a decreased ability to conserve body heat.

◗ Gastrointestinal (GI) problems:
- Aspiration due to poor gag, sucking, and swallowing reflexes caused by a weak esophageal sphincter.
- High caloric and fluid demand with small size but small stomach capacity requiring frequent feedings and supplements.
- Increased metabolic rate and oxygen demands due to energy required for sucking, and low activity tolerance and easy fatigue.
- Limited ability to process nutrients including conversion of amino acids, absorption of fats (low bile salts), or digestion of lactose (needs simple sugars).
- Calcium and phosphorus levels are low because stores are usually built up in the last trimester. Bone demineralization may be noted.
- Decreased tissue perfusion to the GI tract or hypoxemia at birth may result in feeding intolerance and necrotizing enterocolitis.

◑ Decreased renal function:
- Low glomerular filtration rate due to low renal blood flow and hypoxia resulting in oliguria or anuria
- Limited ability of the preterm infant's kidneys to concentrate urine, leading to excretion of excess fluid and risk for dehydration
- Excretion of glucose by the immature kidneys, leading to hypoglycemia
- Decreased ability of the kidneys to buffer, with excess excretion of bicarbonate and resulting metabolic acidosis
- Decreased ability of premature kidneys to excrete drugs, leading to toxicity of drugs at lower levels and high susceptibility to nephrotoxic drugs

◑ Altered immune system:
- High risk for infection because passive immunity gained from mother usually is received by the fetus in the last trimester.
- Preterm skin surface provides less defense against invading organisms.
- IgA, a significant immunoglobulin needed by the newborn that is acquired through breast milk only, does not cross the placenta; thus, the premature newborn must have breast milk to gain this protection.

◑ Neurologic system:
- Myelination of nerves occurs beginning with the second trimester until birth. The closer to term the fetus is, the less disruption of neurologic function is noted.
- Intracranial hemorrhage and intraventricular hemorrhage (with possible hydrocephalus) are the most common complications of preterm infants. The fragile vasculature of the brain easily ruptures in the presence of hypoxia, as commonly occurs with birth asphyxia or birth trauma.
- Preterm newborns have different response patterns than term newborns with fewer reactive periods, decreased responsiveness, and weaker muscle tone. The pattern can be used to determine the best times for feeding and bonding.

TREATMENTS

◑ Radiant warmer or incubator to assist with temperature control.
◑ Dietary support with breast milk and special preterm formula with extra protein and calories. Additional support includes the following:
- A diet high in polyunsaturated fat (well tolerated by preterm newborn)
- Multivitamin supplementation of vitamins A, D, E, and iron
- Calcium, phosphorus, and vitamin D supplements for bone mineralization

- Oral (breast/bottle), naso/orogastric gavage, or total parenteral nutrition provided for nutritional support based on the infant's ability to tolerate nutrition
- ◑ Fluid replacement: There is an increased need for this if radiant warmer is used to maintain temperature.
- ◑ Follow-up treatment for long-term needs:
  - Neurologic deficits, such as lower IQ, seizures, and palsy, are difficult to predict and highly influenced by the family support system and socioeconomic status (resources).
  - Speech deficits.
  - Retinopathy.
  - Bronchopulmonary dysplasia (due to damaged alveoli).
  - Auditory defects.

6 NURSING INTERVENTIONS

- ◑ Support fetal respiratory status, note respiratory distress, and provide oxygen if ordered.
- ◑ Maintain warm environment to prevent cold stress.
- ◑ Initiate feeding as quickly as possible and schedule frequent feedings.
- ◑ Plan activities to avoid fatigue.
- ◑ Encourage contact between the newborn and the parents and family.
- ◑ Monitor the newborn's breath sounds and pulse oximetry.
- ◑ Monitor vital signs.
- ◑ Assess temperature via axillary route every 4 hours.
- ◑ Monitor for skin breakdown.
- ◑ Provide family teaching regarding the need for ongoing monitoring of growth and development with appropriate support for the family and the infant if developmental delay is noted.

SMALL FOR GESTATIONAL AGE (SGA)

5 WHAT WENT WRONG?

A fetus is considered small for its gestational age if its weight is at or less than 10th percentile. The SGA newborn is also described as having experienced intrauterine growth restriction (IUGR) caused by maternal factors, placental factors, or fetal conditions. The major risk factors for SGA include smoking, drug or alcohol use, multiple gestations, gestational hypertension, maternal malnutrition, disease or infection, decreased placental perfusion (such as with a small placenta or placenta previa), fetal infection (such as rubella), or congenital anomalies.

SIGNS AND SYMPTOMS

- ◑ Weight at or below 10th percentile
- ◑ Reduced body dimensions

○ Reduced fetal subcutaneous fat and loose skin
○ Scant scalp hair
○ Signs of hypothermia
○ Decreased muscle mass
○ Flat abdomen
○ Hypoxia, possibly with respiratory distress
○ Umbilical cord that is thin and dry instead of gray, moist, and shiny
○ Wide skull sutures due to poor bone growth

TEST RESULTS

○ Ultrasound may reveal small fetal size for gestational age.
○ Blood glucose may indicate hypoglycemia.
○ Chest X-ray may indicate meconium aspiration.
○ Complete blood count (CBC) may show polycythemia due to fetal hypoxia or fetal stress.
○ Arterial blood gas may indicate chronic hypoxia due to poor placental perfusion.

TREATMENTS

○ Cesarean delivery if there are signs that the fetus cannot tolerate labor
○ Incubator post birth for temperature control if hypothermia is noted
○ Frequent vital signs, blood glucose, and temperature screening
○ Early and frequent feedings (every 3 hours) with supplements or glucose as tolerated

NURSING INTERVENTIONS

○ Support fetal respiratory status through suctioning as needed.
○ Note respiratory distress.
○ Maintain warm environment to prevent cold stress.
○ Initiate feeding as quickly as possible and schedule frequent feedings.
○ Plan activities to avoid fatigue.
○ Encourage contact between the newborn and the parents and family.
○ Preventive care: Includes maternal nutrition education to prevent inadequate weight gain and gestational diabetes.
○ Monitor newborn breath sounds and pulse oximetry.
○ Monitor vital signs.
○ Assess temperature via axillary route every 4 hours.
○ Monitor for skin breakdown.
○ Provide family teaching regarding the need for ongoing monitoring of growth and development with appropriate support for the family and infant if developmental delay is noted.

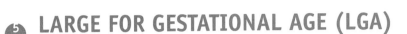

LARGE FOR GESTATIONAL AGE (LGA)

WHAT WENT WRONG?

A fetus is considered excessively large (**macrosomic**) if its weight is above the 90th percentile or exceeds 4,000 g. The primary contributors to macrosomic fetal development are maternal diabetes and post-term pregnancy. A fetus that is LGA is at risk for several conditions:

- Birth injury to fetal clavicles due to **shoulder dystocia** (inability of the fetal shoulder to descend under the maternal symphysis pubis during birth)
- Neonatal hypoglycemia (tremors, seizures, hypotonia, apnea), polycythemia, hyperviscosity, and hypocalcemia: Conditions associated with maternal diabetes
- Erb-Duchenne paralysis secondary to injury at birth

SIGNS AND SYMPTOMS

- Fetal size assessed during Leopold maneuvers indicates LGA.
- Labor **dystocia** (**dysfunctional labor**) is noted with failure of labor to progress.
- FHR may reveal distress during contraction related to shoulder dystocia.
- Newborn will have increased body fat.
- If the infant is from a diabetic mother, cardiomegaly may be noted.

TREATMENTS

- If the infant is of a diabetic mother (IDM) the exposure to excess glucose levels will result in a high production of insulin due to hyperplasia of the pancreatic cells. After maternal glucose supply is removed with birth, hypoglycemia can occur. IV glucose is provided if blood glucose cannot be maintained (>40 mg/dL) with feedings.
- Hypocalcemia, if present, may require treatment with calcium supplement.

NURSING INTERVENTIONS

- Preventive care: Includes maternal nutrition education to prevent excessive weight gain and strict control of gestational diabetes to avoid fetal impact.
- Monitor contraction frequency, duration, and intensity, and note labor progression or lack of labor progression.
- Preparation at time of birth for vacuum-assisted or forceps-assisted birth.
- Assist laboring mother into the lithotomy position to increase pelvic outlet.
- Apply suprapubic pressure during birth to assist mother in bearing down for delivery of fetal shoulder.
- Assess the newborn to detect birth trauma (i.e., clavicle fracture or paralysis).

POSTMATURE NEWBORN

Infants born after 42 weeks of gestation are deemed to be postmature. While these babies may be large for their gestational age, most will be AGA and reveal few symptoms. Postmaturity syndrome may be noted in some newborns who exhibit hypoglycemia due to depletion of glycogen stores, oligohydramnios (decreased amniotic fluid), in utero hypoxia evidenced by meconium aspiration, polycythemia due to increased blood cells in response to hypoxia, and seizures, as well as cold stress due to poor development or loss of subcutaneous fat. The prolonged pregnancy contributes to aging of the placenta with decreased functioning and decreased fetal nutrition and oxygenation.

SIGNS AND SYMPTOMS

- Dry skin; thin, loose, and cracking skin.
- Lack of lanugo or vernix.
- Long fingernails and scalp hair.
- Body is long and thin without fat layers.
- Meconium staining (yellow-green color) of skin and umbilical cord.
- Hypothermia.
- Dyspnea and respiratory distress (if meconium aspiration occurs).

TEST RESULTS

- Blood glucose may show hypoglycemia.
- Temperature may be below normal.
- Hematocrit (central line testing) may reveal polycythemia.

TREATMENTS

- Fluid may be infused in utero to decrease the concentration of meconium-stained amniotic fluid and reduce the impact of meconium aspiration.
- Oxygen support as indicated for respiratory distress.
- Blood glucose monitoring with intravenous glucose to treat hypoglycemia.
- Fluid infusions to reduce viscosity of the blood due to polycythemia.
- Early feeding to support glucose levels.
- Warm environment to compensate for lack of subcutaneous fat.

NURSING INTERVENTIONS

- Preventive care: Includes maternal nutrition education to prevent excessive weight gain and strict control of gestational diabetes to avoid fetal impact.
- Monitor FHR and contraction frequency, duration, and intensity, and note labor progression or lack of labor progression.

- Assess for respiratory distress, hypoglycemia, or other complication upon birth.
- Provide support care: Early feedings with supplements, monitor blood glucose, provide oxygen as ordered for respiratory distress.
- Assess the newborn to detect birth trauma (i.e., clavicle fracture or paralysis) if LGA.
- Support the family and provide teaching on the need for follow-up monitoring for possible long-term problems.

CONCLUSION

Fetal development generally proceeds in an orderly fashion, moving from conception and cell division to the formation of the brain, heart, and other body organs and structures. Early development is critical for structure formation, and late development is important for the full function and maturity of organ systems. Fetal exposure to trauma from toxic substances or unfavorable conditions such as malnutrition or hypoxia can result in damage to the fetus that is irreversible. Key points to remember include the following:

- The stages of fetal growth include the preembryonic stage or germinal period, during which cell duplication and uterine implantation occurs; the embryonic stage, during which the body and extremities are formed; and the fetal stage, which includes the growth of the fetus until birth.
- The length and weight of the embryo and fetus should increase each period with increasing organ function and structure refinement.
- Adipose tissue increases in late pregnancy to provide fat stores and newborn insulation.
- Fetal circulation allows blood to flow from the placenta through the heart, but bypasses the nonfunctioning lungs through openings designed to shunt blood from one side of the heart to the other and out to the fetal body.
- Multiple fetuses proceed through the development process as one fetus does, but maternal nutrients, and in some cases placenta and chorion, are shared, thus placing a higher demand on the mother and increasing the risks for problems in fetal development.
- Rh or ABO incompatibility can cause maternal development of antibodies to the fetal blood. These antibodies can attack the fetal blood, resulting in hemolysis and severe newborn anemia. An Rh immune globulin (RhoGAM) should be given to the unsensitized mother after each pregnancy to prevent antibody production. No preventive treatment is available for ABO incompatibility, and transfusions should be available for the newborn, in case the need arises.
- Teratogens can interfere with fetal development. The earlier the exposure of the developing fetus to the toxin, the more severe the damage that can result.

O Nutritional deficits, hyperthermia, and teratogen exposure can impact varied organs depending upon the stage of fetal development in which the exposure occurs.

O Neural tube defect can occur if incomplete closure occurs with or without spinal cord or meninges protrusion. Nursing care focuses on prevention of injury or infection until repair is performed, then postoperative care for the newborn and family.

O Genetic anomalies can occur secondary to hereditary or chromosomal abnormalities. Extra chromosomes or missing chromosomes can result in alterations in body structure form and function, including altered mental ability.

O Genetic anomalies commonly involve multisystem impacts; some effects may not be evident at birth or in the early infancy period.

O Alterations in fetal growth may occur as a result of preterm birth and intrauterine growth restriction due to maternal, placental, or fetal conditions resulting in a small for gestational age (SGA) newborn; excess exposure to high glucose levels resulting in the birth of a large for gestational age (LGA) newborn; or post-term birth.

O Excess or inadequate gestational time or fetal weight can result in difficulty in fetal tolerance to the birth process as well as complications for the newborn due to altered body system function.

O Nursing care when fetal development alterations are present includes assisting the family in adjusting to the altered newborn function and promoting family support of optimal newborn and child development and management of complications, if applicable.

? FINAL CHECKUP

1. **In what way does fetal circulation differ from newborn circulation?**
   a. The blood flows from the right atria to the right ventricle in fetal circulation but not in newborn circulation.
   b. The blood flows to the lungs from the right atria in fetal circulation.
   c. Blood flow bypasses the lungs and flows to the aorta in fetal circulation.
   d. Blood flow bypasses the aorta and returns to the placenta in newborn circulation.
   e. a and c

2. **Identical twins would result from what pattern of conception?**
   a. Two ova fertilized by two spermatozoa
   b. One ovum fertilized by two separate spermatozoa
   c. Two separate ova fertilized by one spermatozoa
   d. One ovum fertilized by one spermatozoa

3. **Fetal assessment reveals that a 24-week fetus has a length of 15 cm (C-R) and a weight of approximately 400 g. What would the nurse conclude from these findings?**
   a. The fetus is longer than expected for this stage of development.
   b. Intrauterine growth restriction is evident from the findings.
   c. The findings support the risk for the fetus being LGA at birth.
   d. Preparations should be made for a post-term birth for this fetus.

4. **What statement is true about ABO and Rh incompatibility?**
   a. ABO incompatibility is more dangerous in the second pregnancy than the first pregnancy.
   b. Rh incompatibility is not an issue if the pregnancy was terminated in the first trimester.
   c. RhoGAM should be given to the mother after birth to protect her from anemia due to fetal antibodies.
   d. Hemolysis of the fetal blood can occur in pregnancies with ABO or Rh incompatibility.

5. **An ultrasound indicates that the top of the fetal skull is missing. The nurse should identify this as what condition?**
   a. Anencephaly
   b. Cystica meningocele
   c. Occulta
   d. Encephalocele

6. **An amniocentesis is performed and the α-fetoprotein test reveals a low level. The nurse would expect what response from the primary care provider?**
   a. An ultrasound will be ordered to assess the neural tube defect.
   b. The parents will be told of the high likelihood of a neural tube defect.
   c. No further test may be ordered since neural tube defect is not likely.
   d. An abortion will be ordered since the test is positive for anencephaly.

7. **In explaining Down syndrome to parents, the nurse would include what information?**
   a. The underlying genetic defect is a missing trisomy 21 chromosome.
   b. The condition is not likely to cause any lasting effect on the child.
   c. Both trisomy 21 and trisomy 13 are associated with death within the first 3 months of life.
   d. The degree of mental retardation will vary from complete dependence to independence.

8. **An infant is born at 37½ weeks having a weight of 3200 g. The newborn is considered to be in what category?**
   a. Small for gestational age
   b. Large for gestational age
   c. Appropriate for gestational age
   d. Premature with intrauterine growth restriction
   e. Macrosomic with postmaturity

9. **A premature newborn would gain passive immunity through which source of nutrition?**
   a. Fortified bottle formula
   b. Breast feeding on demand
   c. Orogastric gavage formula
   d. Total parenteral nutrition

10. **What condition is most likely to be noted in infants who are SGA or LGA?**
   a. Increased subcutaneous fat
   b. Hypothermia
   c. Hypoglycemia
   d. Decreased subcutaneous fat

ANSWERS

Routine Checkup
   1. c
   2. Undergo prenatal testing for infection and have treatment as soon as possible to prevent the transmission of the infection to the fetus.

Final Checkup

1. c	2. d	3. b	4. d	5. a
6. c	7. d	8. c	9. b	10. c

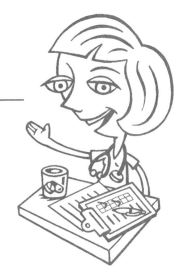

CHAPTER 8

Childbirth Preparation

Objectives

At the end of this chapter, the student will be able to:

1 Assess the level of preparation for the expectant mother and family for the childbearing experience and parenting.

2 Discuss the options in delivery settings, types, attendants, and preparations for labor.

3 Address issues related to cultural beliefs about pregnancy, labor and delivery, and newborn care.

4 Identify nutritional needs of the expectant mother to promote a healthy pregnancy.

5 Describe activities and exercises that will strengthen the maternal body and muscles for a healthy pregnancy and birth.

6 Describe the aspects of birthing programs used to prepare the expectant female and family for the pregnancy, labor and delivery, and newborn parenting process.

KEY TERMS

Anorexia nervosa	Pica
Bulimia nervosa	Pudendal block
Effleurage	Recommended dietary allowance
Epidural block	Spinal block
Maternal parity	

OVERVIEW

The woman and family preparing for the birth of a child face a number of questions and anxieties. To determine the care and learning needs of the woman and family, a thorough assessment is performed, followed by preparation of a plan to provide information and instruction related to the lifestyle adjustments and new skills needed to ensure a healthy pregnancy, birth, and adjustment to parenting a newborn. Issues will range from change in nutritional needs to choice of pain relief measures during the labor process. The family-centered approach requires that the expectant mother and her family or support system be included in the teaching and support provided by the nurse.

ASSESSMENT

1 A prenatal assessment will provide data regarding the expectant mother's general health and any potential problems related to the pregnancy and adjustment to the newborn (including physiologic, socioeconomic, and emotional problems). Several of the issues the pregnant woman will face were discussed with the physiologic changes of pregnancy in Chapter 6. Prenatal care encompasses general health measures, particularly addressing chronic illnesses and nutritional support, needed to maximize maternal health and meet fetal needs. Decision making regarding choices of caregivers, location and type of delivery, and desired comfort measures, in addition to the initial preparation for the care of a newborn, will be addressed during the prenatal period.

PRENATAL CARE

2 The primary location for prenatal care is frequently a community health department, clinic, or doctor's/certified nurse midwife's office. Educational materials are available for the client and family on the Internet, in addition to those provided by the health-care provider. Home health care may be available, and needed, for women who have difficulty accessing health care, and it may also be needed in high-risk pregnancy situations in which bed rest is required.

⓵ Among other client-specific measures, prenatal assessments and care include addressing the following:

- ⓞ Current history of concerns, particularly related to pregnancy.
- ⓞ Assessment data including vital signs, weight, and urine specimen.
- ⓞ Tests for fetal assessment (Doppler pulse, ultrasound, etc.) if indicated. The woman and family may have an initial look at the fetus and hear the fetal heartbeat.
- ⓞ Cervical examination that may be performed, if indicated.
- ⓞ Nutritional habits, pre-pregnancy and current (including craved substances such as starch or dirt/clay), should be assessed as a baseline for nutrition teaching.

⓹ **Care of the father and family** will include explaining the common issues in pregnancy and answering any questions. Using measures such as an empathy belly to help the support individuals understand what the expectant mother may be experiencing so that they can anticipate and better meet maternal needs is an effective strategy. Classes are available for providing the mother and family with information and teaching related to coping with pregnancy and preparation for delivery and newborn care. Determining the readiness of the support system members for the challenges, both physical and emotional, related to pregnancy, and for the onset of labor and the birth experience, allows the nurse to plan appropriate teaching to prepare them. Discussions about the father's and family members' concerns about choices of delivery measures, or more personal issues such as sexual activity during pregnancy or choice of breast-feeding or bottle-feeding of the newborn promotes their involvement in the pregnancy experience and increases support for the expectant woman.

⓺ **Siblings** often have questions and concerns related to pregnancy, the impact of the maternal pregnancy experience and the newborn on the family as a whole, and their role in the new family structure in particular. Prenatal education should allow time for interaction with family members, particularly siblings. Clear communication of needs and expectations helps the siblings and other family members be the needed support resources for the expectant mother and father and promotes healthy family function.

⓷ **Cultural concerns** include addressing practices and beliefs that may be different from those of the health-care provider but are important to the expectant family. Communication difficulties should be anticipated secondary to language barriers, and an interpreter should be provided when indicated. If indicated by cultural norms and patient preference, only female caregivers should be allowed to touch the expectant mother. If culture dictates, and as approved and requested by the mother, the head of the family should be included in information giving and decision-making activities. Unless prohibited by best practice and client safety, cultural preferences and taboos should be acknowledged and adhered to. Assess any substances the expectant mother ingests or is exposed to in order to determine if there may be potential harm to the fetus or mother, and discuss any need to alter or eliminate a specific cultural practice to ensure maternal and fetal safety.

NUTRITION NEEDS

The first trimester may present nutritional concerns due to nausea and vomiting as the mother adjusts to hormone shifts alternating with intense hunger due to fetal nutrition needs. A daily multivitamin regimen may reduce the risk of nutritional deficit due to nausea/vomiting. Alternative medicine used to treat nausea includes ginger, and pyridoxine (vitamin B_6) or over-the-counter antihistamines (with permission of the care provider) may be recommended. A steroid may be used to treat severe nausea and vomiting, but the danger to the fetus often outweighs the benefits. Instruct the woman to notify her health-care provider if vomiting occurs more than once daily or if dehydration (dry lips/mucous membranes, minimal dark urine) occurs. An antiemetic, such as promethazine (Phenergan) may be ordered but should be avoided if possible.

Nutrition assessment should determine issues related to maternal eating including food habits, culture, economics, and knowledge level, as well as willingness to alter habits to maximize health. Additional considerations that may impact nutritional status during pregnancy include the following:

- Nutritional status prior to pregnancy.
- **Maternal parity:** Number and interval between previous pregnancies and outcome of pregnancy will impact maternal nutrition need.
- Maternal age: Adolescent expectant mothers will have growth needs in addition to the increased nutrition needs from the pregnancy. Erratic teen eating habits could result in insufficient nutrients for the mother and fetus. Planning ways to meet nutritional needs while maintaining teen activities with peers (nutritious snacks, healthy choices from fast food menus) will promote compliance with a healthy diet.
- Stage of pregnancy: In early pregnancy rapid cell growth means poor nutritional supply could result in permanent damage to the growing fetus.
- Essential dietary element intake must be increased during pregnancy and lactation. The **recommended dietary allowance** (RDA) and adequate intake (AI) are increased for pregnant and lactating females.

- Maternal weight gain is expected due to the increase in fetal size, amniotic fluid production, uterus expansion, blood volume increase, breast tissue growth, and increased maternal stores.
- Weight gain varies by trimester with the following:
  - 1.6–2.3 kg gain in the first trimester.
  - 0.5 kg/wk weight gain during the second and third trimesters.
  - Weight gain is a little higher for underweight women.
  - Weight gain should be lower (0.3 kg/wk) for overweight women.
  - In a multiple fetus pregnancy, weight gain is higher (0.7 kg/wk for twins).
- Insufficient maternal weight gain has been noted to result in preterm birth and related newborn distress, and small-for-gestational-age/low-birth-weight babies.
- Maternal obesity can predispose the pregnant mother to a higher risk of pregnancy-related complications, such as spontaneous abortion, preeclampsia, and diabetes, in addition to increasing the risk for fetal abnormalities. In addition, children of obese mothers are more likely to be obese. Weight gain should be monitored carefully since obesity predisposes a woman to excessive weight gain during pregnancy. Maternal obesity and excessive weight gain are associated with large-for-gestational-age (LGA) babies. Low-calorie diets are not encouraged during pregnancy for obese women since adequate intake is necessary for fetal health. Instead, the desired weight gain is modified and a healthy diet is encouraged with a variety of foods from the food pyramid.
- On average, calories should be increased 300 kcal/day during the second and third trimesters. Carbohydrates and protein intake are increased slightly, and fat should remain no more than 30% of the daily intake.
- Mineral intake should be increased to meet maternal and fetal needs:
  - Calcium and phosphorus are needed for fetal bone and teeth mineralization. If an adequate supply is not available, the mother might suffer deficits as the needs of the fetus are met.
  - Iodine (to prevent cretinism occurrence) is needed in acceptable amounts. An adequate supply is provided through the use of iodized salt.
  - Sodium is needed for metabolism and fluid regulation. Adequate intake is seldom problematic, and excessive sodium should be avoided through elimination of high-salt snacks and added salt as food is eaten.
  - Zinc is needed for protein metabolism and DNA/RNA synthesis. Meat, poultry, seafood, whole grains, and legumes should be consumed to provide dietary zinc.
  - Magnesium is needed for cellular metabolism. Milk, whole grains, dark green vegetables, nuts, and legumes should be consumed to provide dietary magnesium.

- Iron needs increase significantly during pregnancy to provide for fetal and maternal production of blood cells. Iron deficiency anemia can result from low iron stores and the high demand for iron during pregnancy. Lean meats; dark green, leafy vegetables; eggs; and whole grain or enriched bread or cereals. as well as dried fruits, legumes, shellfish, and molasses are good sources of iron. Iron supplements are often prescribed, but the gastrointestinal (GI) distress from iron may make iron supplements difficult to maintain. The use of iron salt could provide the needed increase in iron while reducing sodium from regular salt use to season food.

Nurse Alert **Milk and caffeine may interfere with iron absorption, so supplements should be taken with water.**

- Support to minimize GI distress by recommending the mother eat vegetables and fruit to minimize constipation.
- Vitamins: ADEK, fat-soluble vitamins, are critical for cell growth, night vision, and fetal eye development. Danger lies in excessive ADEK intake, thus monitoring is important. Symptoms of vitamin E and K excess include nausea and GI upset; dry, cracked skin; and hair loss. Symptoms of vitamin D toxicity include thirst, appetite loss, vomiting, weight loss, irritability, weight loss, and high blood calcium levels. Vitamin E is an antioxidant and beneficial for enzymatic and metabolic reactions; however, excessive vitamin E has been associated with newborn coagulation abnormalities. Thus supplements for vitamins ADEK must be used carefully.
- Water-soluble vitamins (vitamin C, B vitamins, and folic acid) are important for the formation of connective tissue and vasculature (vitamin C); coenzyme factors such as cell regulation, glucose oxidation, and energy metabolism (vitamins B_1, B_2, B_6, and B_{12}); and growth, reproduction, and lactation, as well as prevention of megaloblastic anemia (folic acid). The need for these vitamins increases with the need for increased calories and energy.
- Vegetarians, including lacto-ovo vegetarians (who include milk, dairy, and eggs in their vegetable/fruit diet) or vegans who eat no meat or animal byproducts, must watch their diets closely to ensure adequate provision of protein, B vitamins, and sufficient calories since vegetables are filling and low in calories, so total caloric intake could be insufficient for the needs of pregnancy. Additional calcium and vitamin D supplements may be prescribed to ensure adequate supply.

Nurse Alert **Caution mothers to avoid fish and shellfish that are high in mercury and to eat small portions of seafood that is low in mercury. Artificial sweeteners that have clearance through the Food and Drug Administration (FDA) are safe for use by the pregnant woman. Foods might contain salmonella, listeriosus (bacterium found in refrigerated substances such as unpasteurized milk, and some meat, poultry, and seafood), or hepatitis E (particularly in raw meat); thus, proper cleaning and cooking temperatures are critical.**

Eating disorders such as binge and purge eating (bulimia nervosa), or severely limited food intake due to altered self-image as being fat (anorexia nervosa), can result in insufficient caloric intake and threaten the health of the child. Pica (intake of nonfoods such as clay or dirt due to cravings) can also result in inadequate food intake as well as iron deficiency anemia if iron absorption is disrupted. The nurse must be nonjudgmental and work with the family to avoid cultural practices that place the mother or fetus in jeopardy.

Key points in maternal nutrition include the following:

- The woman should eat regularly, 3 regular meals or 6 small meals each day.
- The mother should eat a well-balanced, nutritious diet with a variety of foods that provide the recommended dietary allowance of nutrients adjusted for age and maternal size. Additional calories and nutrients are needed if multiple fetuses are present.
- Inadequate weight gain can result in a small-for-gestational-age infant, and excessive weight gain can result in excessively large newborn size and weight.
- Fruit and vegetables provide fiber in the diet and will reduce the incidence of constipation.
- Iron-rich foods will increase maternal and fetal iron stores.
- A daily multivitamin is prescribed to ensure that needed nutrients are provided.
- Weight loss dieting is prohibited to avoid reducing nutrients to the fetus.
- Adolescent females require additional nutrients for maternal growth as well as fetal development.
- Monitor dietary intake and provide counseling to avoid intake of clay, starch, or other craved nonfood substances (pica), which will reduce needed nutritional intake.
- Monitor laboratory tests that indicate adequacy of nutrition, such as hematocrit and hemoglobin.
- Vegetarians must choose foods to avoid the potential for low protein, iron, zinc, vitamin B_{12}, and calcium since meat and animal products are the usual sources of these nutrients.
- Cultural preferences should be respected when planning a diet for the pregnant female.

ACTIVITY

Exercise provides multiple benefits for the female during pregnancy. The balance of activity and rest is important to reap the benefits and avoid exhaustion or harm from high-risk activity. Specific added exercises for the abdominal and pelvic muscles can be beneficial in preparation for labor and delivery.

- Exercise should be regular, half an hour each day.
- Low impact exercise reduces pressure on the trunk that may be caused by weight-bearing exercises such as jogging.
- Swimming or walking provides good cardiovascular benefits and stress relief.
- Hydration is important, particularly in hot weather. Drink water regularly and avoid getting overheated or excessively tired.
- If unable to talk while exercising, slow the pace and intensity to remain within a comfortable level.
- Do not use a hot tub or sauna, which could cause vasodilation and result in cardiovascular compromise with hypotension and fainting.
- Do not exercise alone. In the event of complications or injury, assistance may be needed.
- Kegel exercises help to strengthen the pelvic muscles used in bearing down during delivery.
- Back exercises, including the pelvic tilt, are beneficial in reducing back pain common to pregnancy.

Activity during labor and prior to birth may include ambulating, sitting in a rocking chair, showering or bathing, or sitting or lying on the bed. If the membrane has ruptured, and the fetus is not engaged, ambulation may be limited to prevent cord prolapse.

✔ ROUTINE CHECKUP 1

1. Why might home health care be indicated in the care of a pregnant woman?

Answer:

2. What represents an appropriate strategy to address a nutritional concern of pregnancy?
   a. Ginger for urinary frequency
   b. Vitamin B_6 for appetite suppression
   c. Increased carbohydrates to meet caloric needs
   d. Low-protein diet in second and third trimesters

Answer:

CHILDBIRTH/DELIVERY OPTIONS

6 When the expectant mother and family begin to adjust to the concept of pregnancy, decisions are made about the plan for childbirth. There are many options for an uncomplicated delivery, and even when a surgical delivery must be performed, there are often options regarding some aspects of the experience, for example, the timing, degree of sedation, and presence of support persons. The expectant mother and family will work with the primary care provider and the nurse to determine the delivery experience that best fits their family, community resources, and in some cases insurance plan or economic resources.

2 The expectant mother and family may choose the traditional hospital ward for labor and delivery, a birthing center, or some may choose to deliver at home. Many hospitals have labor rooms and separate delivery rooms that are similar to operating rooms. Some hospital facilities have regular patient rooms that are equipped to support labor and delivery, as well as the postpartum mother with a newborn living in the room with her. The birthing room may be decorated like a bedroom at home, and a birthing bed or birthing chair may be present for use. The facility may allow for the support person to sleep in the room as well. In some facilities, large baths are available for a water birth, if desired by the expectant mother and family.

Positions for delivery may vary based on the preference of the mother, recommendations from the health-care provider, and facilities available to support position choice. Generally, any position that allows gravity to help the descent of the fetus is acceptable, so the preference of the mother will generally dominate. Positions during birth may include kneeling, squatting, lying on her side, lying on her back on a birthing bed, sitting up in a birthing chair, or positioned on hands and knees. A woman may change positions multiple times prior to the actual birth of the child.

PAIN MANAGEMENT

Because any medication that enters the mother's bloodstream usually enters the fetal system and affects the fetus, the choice of pain relief measure during delivery is a critical one. Some mothers choose to have a natural delivery without medication. Alternative measures are used to minimize discomfort and support is used to help the mother cope with the pain of labor during the delivery. Varied approaches to birth are available:

- Leboyer is an approach to delivery that focuses on minimizing the trauma of fetal transition to extrauterine life by providing a calming environment. Water births are included in the strategies used.
- **6** The Bradley method uses abdominal breathing and general relaxation, promotes partner involvement and support for the mother, and emphasizes natural childbirth without medication. The Dick-Read method uses controlled

breathing with partner support and progressive relaxation to consciously relax all muscles except the uterus for a less stressful labor. The Lamaze method focuses on partner-coached breathing and panting with relaxation using a focal point for concentration during labor. Relaxation is a key element in most childbirth methods and aids in pain relief measures because anxiety and muscle tension can increase the pain experienced by the mother.

Some measures used for pain management include the following:

- **Effleurage:** Light stroking of the abdomen in a circular pattern with the fingertips by the woman or a support person.
- Deep pressure over the back can relieve back discomfort.
- Relaxation exercises: Lying down and progressively tightening and relaxing body parts from head to toe. Variations include touch relaxation, which involves the support person providing comforting touch; and disassociation relaxation, which involves exercises that help the woman focus contractions on one body part (uterus) while relaxing other body parts.
- Breathing exercises are taught to the mother to promote effective oxygenation of the mother and fetus during labor by controlling rapid, irregular breathing due to pain. Deep breathing can also increase relaxation, focus the woman, and distract her from the pain as she performs this task. It also helps the woman to regain a sense of control at a time when she may feel powerless against the labor.
- **Pharmacologic pain intervention** may include a variety of approaches. The mother should understand the medication being provided, the effect of the medication, the impact of the medication on the fetus, alternatives, and associated safety instructions such as sitting up slowly or remaining in bed to avoid an accidental fall.
    - **Epidural block:** Involves injection of anesthesia into the epidural space, which blocks pain reception from the lower body, thus blocking the pains of labor. Opioids may be injected as well to control the pain.

 Nurse Alert **Provide fluids prior to epidural placement and monitor for maternal hypotension, which might occur. Contraindications to an epidural include infection at the site of needle puncture, blood coagulopathies, increased intracranial pressure, medication allergy, or maternal hypotension. Epidural block may be given as an infusion regulated to control for pain. If pain occurs even with continuous infusion (breakthrough pain), additional pain medication may be needed.**

- **Spinal block** involves the anesthesia agent being injected into the spinal fluid. This can be used for a vaginal or cesarean birth. Rapid pain control is achieved; however, hypotension can occur leading to fetal compromise from hypoxia.

Nurse Alert The mother cannot feel the uterine contraction or the urge to push after a spinal block, so the nurse must monitor contractions and instruct the mother when to bear down. If the mother is unable to push, forceps may be needed to assist in the delivery of the baby.

- **Combined spinal-epidural block** can reduce the total level of medication introduced into the maternal system but allow for greater mobility by the laboring woman.
- **Pudendal block** is injection of anesthesia transvaginally to block the pain signal from the pudendal nerve, resulting in relief from pain from the structures in the pelvic region. Pain from uterine contractions is still felt. Maternal hypotension does not occur and no fetal impact is noted, but hematoma, sciatic nerve trauma, or rectal perforation may occur.
- **Local anesthesia:** Usually injected at the time of delivery to allow for episiotomy with minimal discomfort.
- **General anesthesia:** May be needed for cesarean delivery, but the impact is great on the fetus, thus this method is avoided with a high-risk fetus.
- **Systemic pain medication** may be administered during labor to reduce maternal discomfort and promote rest between contractions. Many systemic medications cross the placental barrier and thus will impact the fetus. Since liver function affects the metabolism of the medication, the dose provided to the fetus will remain for a period of time due to the fetus' immature liver function. Opiate-based medications are avoided if the mother has a history of or is suspected to have drug dependence. Guidelines in the use of systemic medication, if the mother provides informed consent, include the following:
- **Maternal and fetal statuses are stable:**
  - Maternal vital signs are within normal range.
  - Fetal heart rate (FHR) is 110–160 bpm with variability and no late decelerations.
  - Fetus is at term and demonstrating acceleration with movement.
- Medication should be administered after labor is well established with adequate dilation and effacement of the cervix and regular contractions. If provided too soon, labor can be lengthened. If the pain medication is provided too late, it will be less beneficial for the mother and will result in the birth of a sedated newborn.
- One side effect of pain medications is sedation. This can help the mother to relax and rest between contractions; however, the medication and side effect is also passed to the fetus, thus effort is made to use the smallest amount possible to allow maximum maternal comfort with minimum fetal sedation and minimum decrease of labor progression. Maternal vital signs, FHR, cervical status (dilation, position, effacement, consistency), and contraction pattern are assessed prior to and after medication is given.

- Most medications are opiate based and can cause dizziness and hypotension, so safety requires bed rest with the side rails raised for injury prevention.
- Urinary retention is caused by some medications, so urinary output and bladder assessments should be performed. Medications include the following:

Medication	Side Effects	Nursing Intervention
Fentanyl (Sublimaze): short-acting—does not cross placental barrier	Neonatal depression, but less than with Demerol; maternal bradycardia, hypotension, muscle rigidity, nausea, and pruritus possible	Monitor maternal response to medication, particularly pulse and respirations; monitor FHR for decrease
Meperidine (Demerol)	Respiratory depression, maternal and fetal, common; fetal sedation possible; maternal constipation, dizziness, and itching possible	Monitor maternal respirations and FHR for signs of depression; if needed provide respiratory support
Nalbuphine hydrochloride (Nubain)	Abdominal cramps and pain, hypotension, bradycardia, blurred vision	Assess pulse and blood pressure— contraindicated if hypersensitivity noted, if allergy attack noted, or bradycardia or hypotension
Butorphanol (Stadol)	Drowsiness common; dizziness, fainting, hypotension possible	Monitor for bladder distention; store away from light and at room temperature

 ROUTINE CHECKUP 2

1. Why should a pregnant client avoid some pain medications?

Answer:

2. Why would a sitting position be more advantageous than a lying position during delivery?
   a. Increased circulation to the head when sitting helps mood during delivery.
   b. Depressed respirations in the sitting position are further depressed when lying down.
   c. Gravity will facilitate fetal descent when sitting during delivery.
   d. Lying down lowers the capacity of the blood to carry oxygen.

Answer:

CHILDBIRTH CLASSES

Prenatal education is critical to assist the expectant female and family in understanding and coping with the pregnancy and delivery experience, and in preparation for care of a newborn. The nurse's role includes assessment of knowledge, planning needed, teaching, and referral to childbirth classes for experiences to prepare the woman and support persons for labor and delivery. Prenatal education should include the following:

- Changes during pregnancy and accompanying discomforts.
- Preventative and relief measures to maximize maternal comfort.
- Diet and exercise planning to promote a healthy pregnancy and a positive labor and delivery process.
- Previous birth experience could impact maternal learning needs positively or negatively depending on the type of experience. Do not assume that the mother knows everything because of previous pregnancy.
- If prior experience was negative, reassure the mother that every experience proceeds differently and address any concerns. The pregnancy experience can vary if maternal factors, such as age, weight, or even mental attitude, are different. Multiple fetuses or complications of pregnancy can cause major differences in pregnancy.
- Stress positive behaviors such as proper diet, exercise, and regular prenatal care.
- Discuss the need to avoid medications and supplements unless approved by a health-care provider.
- Discuss the importance of avoiding alcohol, tobacco, or substance abuse to reduce the risk of birth defects, fetal addiction, a low-birth-weight infant, or other complications.
- Instruct the mother and family regarding complications to monitor for and what to report to the physician/certified nurse midwife.
- Review the prenatal care needed and what will occur during visits, as well as the frequency of visits needed as the pregnancy progresses to later stages.
- Discuss fetal monitoring measures, including ultrasound and amniocentesis, if indicated.
- Genetic counseling is introduced if indicated by maternal or paternal history or age extremes.
- The decision to breast-feed or bottle-feed is made during this prenatal period.
- Childbirth classes discuss issues such as:
  - Method of delivery available (water birth, etc.).
  - Comfort measures during labor (use of medications, epidural, etc.) and their impact on the fetus.
  - Monitoring of fetal movement. Count movements daily for a full minute. Report if they reduce to less than 3 per hour or if movement is not noted for 12 hours.

- Alternate methods to minimize pain, and using distraction techniques and breathing exercises.
- Signs of impending labor.
- Braxton-Hicks contractions versus true labor.
- The labor and delivery process.
- Contact with the infant immediately after delivery.
- Postdelivery care.
- Newborn care and parenting skills.
- Discuss the emotional changes of pregnancy for the mother and family, including siblings.
- Allow verbalization of concerns and ambivalence without demonstrating judgment, and reassure the mother that feelings will shift many times during pregnancy and that hormonal levels will impact emotions at times.
- Journaling may be helpful for working through feelings.

PREPARATION FOR CESAREAN DELIVERY

Increasing numbers of women are requesting cesarean births. Therefore, prenatal teaching includes education on this delivery process. Explanations should be given about the following:

- Incision used and choices allowed, if any
- Anesthesia used for delivery and pain control postpartum
- What sensations will be experienced?
- Ability of the mother to be alert and aware during the birth
- Presence of the father or support person being allowed during the birth
- Videotaping or picture-taking during the birth or in the recovery room
- Delayed instillation of infant eye drops to allow infant-parent bonding
- Physical contact with the infant by the mother (and father/support person) after birth
- Breast-feeding in the recovery area
- Preparatory procedures (including preoperative testing and teaching)
- Postoperative care related to the birth and surgical procedure
- Impact of the surgical procedure on interaction with newborn and family
- Recovery period anticipated

If the cesarean is an emergency the preparation time is limited, but many concerns can be anticipated and addressed. Focus on the reason for the cesarean delivery, the support that will be present, the ability to experience the birth and interact with the newborn (if no fetal distress results), and sensations that might be experienced. Support persons should be included in teaching and be allowed to remain with the woman through experience.

CONCLUSION

Preparation of the expectant mother and family for the pregnancy, birth, and parenting experience provides the basis for a healthy delivery and positive family transition to newborn care. Key points discussed in the chapter include the following:

- A family-centered approach to childbirth preparation involves education and support for the expectant mother and family, including siblings.
- Assessment should include maternal health and habits that may impact the pregnancy, support systems, and the knowledge of the mother and family, as well as concerns.
- Cultural beliefs and practices related to the pregnancy and delivery should be respected and complied with when no danger to the mother or fetus is present.
- Nutrition is critical for the mother and fetus to promote healthy fetal growth and development without harm to the maternal nutrition status. Increased amounts of key nutrients should be ingested daily to support fetal development.
- Adolescent pregnancy presents challenges to nutritional support and requires planning and teaching to support adolescent and fetal growth and development needs.
- Desirable maternal weight gain is adjusted based on age, pre-pregnancy weight, and number of fetuses. Inadequate or excessive weight gain should be avoided due to risk factors for preterm birth, restricted or excessive fetal growth, or maternal complications. A well-balanced meal plan with 3 to 6 meals per day is optimal.
- Eating disorders and nonfood cravings can compromise maternal nutritional intake and fetal nutrition. Teaching and, if needed, referral for counseling should be provided to guide the mother to optimal nutrition.
- Exercise can be beneficial for the expectant mother for stress relief, health maintenance, back pain reduction, and in preparation for labor and delivery.
- Activity should be moderate and low impact, and caution should be taken to avoid fatigue and injury. Ambulation is limited after the membranes rupture to avoid cord prolapse.
- Multiple delivery options exist and maternal and family preference, in addition to available resources and health considerations, will impact the delivery choice.
- Pain management is an important aspect of promoting an effective and positive labor and delivery experience. Use of non-pharmacologic measures, in addition to pharmacologic measures, can provide the most effective and beneficial pain control for the mother with minimal negative

impact on the fetus. Monitor for side effects of some spinal and other nerve blocks and minimize when possible with hydration.

- ◐ Childbirth classes are beneficial for the preparation of the expectant mother and family, including siblings, for the pregnancy and delivery.
- ◐ Preparation of the mother and family for cesarean delivery will promote a positive postoperative and postpartum outcome for the mother, fetus, and family, and reduce anxiety for all involved.

? FINAL CHECKUP

1. **Michelle, age 28, has indicated that since this is her first child she wants to have her pain controlled with a spinal block and a little sedation for her anxiety, but she wants to be awake for the experience. Which childbirth method would not be appropriate for her?**
   a. Lamaze
   b. Bradley
   c. Dick-Read
   d. Leboyer

2. **The nurse should instruct a pregnant client to report which symptom immediately?**
   a. Bleeding from the vagina
   b. Swelling of the feet and ankles
   c. Indigestion after meals
   d. Breast swelling and tenderness

3. **Which statement describes the mineral intake needs during pregnancy?**
   a. Calcium and phosphorus will be provided to the maternal body before meeting fetal needs.
   b. High-salt snacks should be eaten to ensure adequate sodium is ingested.
   c. Iron should be taken with milk to promote absorption into the bloodstream.
   d. Zinc is found in meat and poultry and is needed for protein metabolism.

4. **Which mother would the nurse be most concerned about?**
   a. The woman who gains 2.2 kg by the end of her first trimester.
   b. The woman who gains 1.5 kg per week in the third trimester.
   c. The woman who gains 2.0 kg in 1 month of the second trimester.
   d. The woman who gains 0.5 kg each week of the second trimester.

5. **India Ires, an expectant mother, states it is her family's custom to place a stuffed snake head at the bedside during the labor process to ward off bad spirits and asks to place it on the bedside table. How should the nurse respond?**
   a. "The doctor does not allow any foreign objects in the room during labor."
   b. "The room must be kept sterile during labor and delivery, but your family can bring it in after the baby is born."
   c. "That is fine. Let me know if there is anything you need to position the snake head on the table as your custom requires."
   d. "There are no bad spirits here so you don't have to worry, we have a positive staff."

6. **Vegetarians who eat no animal byproducts are at highest risk for what nutrient deficit?**
   a. B vitamin
   b. Vitamin C
   c. Sodium
   d. Iodine

7. **Which activity would be beneficial for an expectant mother?**
   a. A vigorous jog around the block each morning to increase circulation
   b. Soaking in a hot tube for a half hour to relax pelvic muscles
   c. Pelvic tilt exercises to loosen pelvic joints to ease fetal descent
   d. Kegel exercises to strengthen maternal pelvic muscles

8. **What statement by a pregnant woman would indicate the need for additional education?**
   a. "I should avoid smoking and being around people who are smoking."
   b. "I need to eat dark green vegetables and meat or fish for protein."
   c. "I can decrease constipation by avoiding vegetables and fruit."
   d. "I should avoid tea and coffee when I am taking my iron tablet."

9. **A laboring woman who received a dose of fentanyl (Sublimaze) for the pain states she is feeling less pain but is concerned because she is also very sleepy. How should the nurse respond?**
   a. "The medication is probably too strong for you, I will get the antidote."
   b. "I will monitor you closely so let me know if the sleepiness decreases."
   c. "Lie quietly and I will notify the doctor about this medication reaction."
   d. "Sedation is expected and should help you to rest between contractions."

10. **What medication should the nurse question if ordered for a laboring female who has a history of hypertension?**
   a. Fentanyl (Sublimaze)
   b. Butorphanol (Stadol)
   c. Nalbuphine hydrochloride (Nubain)
   d. Meperidine (Demerol)

ANSWERS

Routine Checkup 1

1. If a woman is in a high risk situation and requires bed rest, home health care may be indicated.
2. c

Routine Checkup 2

1. Because any medication that enters the maternal system affects the fetus, and because some pain medications can cause the symptoms of some chronic conditions to increase.
2. c

Final Checkup

1. b	2. a	3. d	4. b	5. c
6. a	7. d	8. c	9. d	10. b

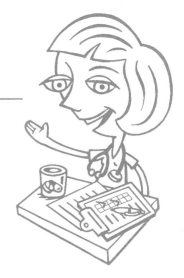

CHAPTER **9**

Complications of Pregnancy

Objectives

At the end of this chapter, the student will be able to:

1. Identify conditions and circumstances that may result in a pregnancy complication.

2. Discuss assessments and diagnostic findings related to complications of pregnancy.

3. Discuss care and treatment regimens associated with each complication of pregnancy.

4. Determine appropriate nursing interventions associated with each complication of pregnancy.

5. Teach and support parents and families regarding the care required to minimize mortality and morbidity secondary to complications of pregnancy.

 KEY TERMS

Gestational trophoblastic disease	Parity
Gravidity	Salpingostomy
HELLP syndrome	Thrombocytopenia
Macrosomia	Tocolysis

OVERVIEW

Complications of pregnancy can occur at any stage, beginning with fertilization and through birth. Early diagnosis of a risk factor for a complication or the early onset of the complication can lead to early treatment and prevention of damage to the mother or fetus.

Often the cause of the complication is not known, but many associated conditions can provide an opportunity to anticipate the condition and prevent or minimize the negative consequences.

ECTOPIC PREGNANCY (EP)

WHAT WENT WRONG?

In ectopic pregnancy the sperm fertilizes the ovum, but the transition from the fallopian tube to the uterus is interrupted and the zygote is implanted outside of the uterus, usually in the tube. The causes may vary but any condition that results in damage to the tubes including pelvic inflammatory disease (PID), endometriosis, prior surgery, exposure to diethylstilbestrol (DES), or the presence of an intrauterine device (IUD) could contribute to ectopic pregnancy. Prognosis is poor for the embryo, which cannot grow to term, and guarded for the mother if the ectopic pregnancy is not terminated before the tube ruptures and hemorrhage occurs.

SIGNS AND SYMPTOMS

- Missed menses.
- Sudden lower quadrant stabbing pain on one side of the abdomen.
- Vaginal bleeding may or may not be present: Scant dark spotting (may indicate rupture has occurred; however, bleeding into the peritoneum may occur in some cases).
- Symptoms of early pregnancy may be reported: Breast changes, nausea, etc.
- Nausea and vomiting may increase if rupture occurs.
- Shoulder pain may be reported: Referred pain from irritation of the diaphragm or phrenic nerve by blood.
- Hypotension, tachycardia, and pallor may be noted if rupture occurs secondary to bleeding and shock.

TEST RESULTS

- Hemoglobin and hematocrit may be low if bleeding occurs.
- Human chorionic gonadotropin (hCG) is elevated, confirming pregnancy.
- Progesterone level is elevated.
- Ultrasound reveals an empty womb.
- White blood cell (WBC) count elevated.

➌ TREATMENTS

- ◑ Methotrexate is administered to stop cell division and enlargement of the zygote to prevent fallopian tube rupture and spare the fallopian tube.
- ◑ **Salpingostomy** (surgical excision of a portion of or entire fallopian tube)
  - Linear salpingostomy to remove unruptured ectopic pregnancy and save the fallopian tube
  - Laproscopic salpingostomy to remove entire tube (if rupture has occurred)

 Drug Alert **Side effects of methotrexate include stomatitis and suppression of blood cell production, thus monitor for oral lesions, anemia, thrombocytopenia, bleeding, and infection.**

 Nurse Alert **Instruct the client that birth control should be used while on methotrexate, and caution the client that hair loss will occur and to prepare for alternate styles to maintain self-esteem.**

➍ NURSING INTERVENTIONS

- ◑ Monitor the client closely for signs of ectopic pregnancy to facilitate early diagnosis and treatment.
- ◑ Monitor vital signs for symptoms of rupture:
  - Blood pressure, pulse, respirations, and temperature
  - Urine output
  - Skin color
- ◑ Replace fluid loss.

 Drug Alert **Assess for signs of adverse reaction to methotrexate—dizziness, seizures, nausea and vomiting, gastrointestinal (GI) hemorrhage, anemia, urinary retention, renal failure, lung disease, etc.**

- **Prepare client for surgery.**

 Nurse Alert **Patient Education:** ➎ **Reinforce the explanation of ectopic pregnancy and support the family in the adjustment to the lost pregnancy (if indicated).**

- **Provide postoperative care for abdominal surgery or laparoscopic surgery.**

➎ **Cultural Considerations:** Some cultures may consider the ectopic pregnancy to be the death of a child and may require that the zygote and tube be disposed of in a special manner. Be alert to this possible need and accommodate the family if possible.

HYPEREMESIS GRAVIDARUM

⚠ WHAT WENT WRONG?

Nausea and vomiting secondary to elevated hCG becomes extreme. Nausea and vomiting is prolonged beyond 12 weeks of pregnancy and causes weight loss of 5% or more from the woman's weight prior to pregnancy. Dehydration, electrolyte imbalance, ketosis, and acetonuria may also result from the continued vomiting. Persistent decreased nutrients to the fetus can result in restricted growth of the fetus and possible preterm birth. Liver dysfunction may be noted with the condition.

⚠ SIGNS AND SYMPTOMS

- ◐ History may reveal risk factors:
  - First pregnancy
  - Pregnant woman less than 20 years of age
  - Obese pregnant woman
  - Multiple birth pregnancy
  - History of psychiatric disorder
  - Hyperthyroidism
  - Vitamin B deficiencies
  - Elevated stress level
  - **Gestational trophoblastic disease:** Growth and degeneration of cells in the placenta to grape-like clusters—complete mole with no fetus or partial mole with genetic material derived from fertilized ovum
- ◐ Vomiting over a prolonged period
- ◐ Dehydration: Poor skin turgor, dry mucous membranes
- ◐ Weight loss
- ◐ Hypotension
- ◐ Tachycardia

⚠ TEST RESULTS

- ◐ Urinalysis reveals ketones, acetones, and an elevated specific gravity.
- ◐ Electrolyte imbalances: Reduced sodium, potassium, and chloride.
- ◐ Acidosis due to vomiting of bases.
- ◐ Elevated liver enzymes.
- ◐ Thyroid test shows elevated levels.
- ◐ Hematocrit may be elevated due to dehydration and hemoconcentration.

⚠ TREATMENTS

- ◐ Fluid therapy as needed to maintain hydration: Ringer's lactate.
- ◐ Electrolyte replacement as indicated.
- ◐ Vitamin B_6 and other vitamins as indicated.

- Antiemetic (promethazine or metoclopramide) to control nausea and vomiting.
- Nothing by mouth (npo) for 24 to 48 hours.
- Advance diet if no vomiting within 24 hours to 6 small meals.
- Enteral nutrition by feeding tube or total parental nutrition if vomiting persists.

NURSING INTERVENTIONS

- Support the woman and family by explaining and answering questions.
- Provide dry toast, crackers, or cereal when solid food is permitted.
- Monitor the mother's intake and output closely to judge return of hydration or continued fluid imbalance.
- Review and monitor the woman for common adverse effects of promethazine (including dizziness, constipation, urinary retention) or metoclopramide (including dizziness, sleeplessness, dystonia).

 Nurse Alert **Review history for conditions in which this drug is contraindicated, including seizure disorder, breast cancer, or GI obstruction. Hold drug and report to primary care provider/physician.**

Patient Safety: Assess mental status for signs of depression, anxiety, or irritability, which may indicate adverse reactions to the medication.

PREMATURE RUPTURE OF MEMBRANES (PROM)/ PRETERM PROM (PPROM)

WHAT WENT WRONG?

Spontaneous rupture of the membranes prior to the onset of labor is considered premature rupture. If this occurs prior to 37 weeks gestation it is considered preterm. The cause is unknown, but associated conditions include multiple pregnancy, infection (including urinary tract infection), incompetent cervix, history of laser conization, genital tract anomalies in the mother, hemorrhage during pregnancy, prior history of PPROM, hydramnios, amniocentesis, placenta previa, abruption placentae, or trauma. If not prevented or treated quickly, maternal injury could include chorioamnionitis—infection of the amniotic fluid—or endometritis or more severe morbidity and possible mortality; fetal consequences could include premature birth with respiratory distress syndrome due to immature lungs, fetal sepsis due to exposure to pathogen, umbilical cord prolapse or compression, or malpresentation. The earlier the occurrence of PROM, the greater the possibility of severe morbidity or mortality.

SIGNS AND SYMPTOMS

- Passage of fluid from the vagina—clear/blood-tinged amniotic fluid—confirmed by a positive nitrazine paper test (dark blue).
- Cervical dilation possible with effacement and fetal descent possible if preterm birth imminent.
- Signs of infection may be present (fever, foul odor to discharge, fetal and maternal tachycardia).
- Preterm labor may be present with preterm premature rupture of membrane (PPROM).
- If cord descends signs of prolapsed cord may be present (see condition).

TEST RESULTS

- Sterile speculum examination reveals amniotic fluid in the vagina, confirmed by a positive nitrazine paper test (dark blue) and a microscopic examination (ferning test).

Nurse Alert **Avoid digital examination to prevent introduction of pathogens to fetus and mother.**

- **Fetal monitoring is continued and may show no distress initially.**
- **Cultures may reveal infection or initially may be negative.**
- **Newborn is assessed for sepsis and prophylactic antibiotics may be given.**
- **Ultrasound may reveal gestational age, amniotic fluid remaining, and fetal status.**

TREATMENTS

- Conservative treatment of PROM if pregnancy is less than 37 weeks gestation to prolong the pregnancy for fetal maturity.
  - Bed rest, hospitalization.
  - Fetal lung maturity testing as the fetus approaches 34 weeks.
  - Corticosteroids to promote fetal lung maturity.
  - Fetal monitoring for first hours post-rupture.
  - Nonstress tesing (NST) is continued to monitor the fetus.
- Antibiotics may be given if infection is suspected or confirmed.
- Fetus is delivered vaginally or by cesarean if symptoms of infection are noted.

NURSING INTERVENTIONS

- Encourage the woman to lie on her left side to promote optimal uterine and placental perfusion.
- Question the woman concerning the time of rupture and onset of labor (if present) to determine the length of time without barrier to pathogens.

- Monitor maternal vital signs and fetal heart rate every 4 hours or more frequently if abnormalities are noted.
- Monitor WBC count, temperature, pulse rate, and the nature of amniotic fluid for signs of infection.
- Support the woman and her partner and prepare for possible early birth.

PRETERM LABOR (PTL)

WHAT WENT WRONG?

Labor that begins between 20 and 36 weeks of pregnancy is termed preterm labor. Conditions that seem to contribute to preterm labor include abnormal cervical length, prior history of preterm birth or preterm labor, infection, or cervicovaginal fibronectin (fetal protein not normally found in vaginal tract after 22 weeks, which is a high predictor for preterm labor). If preterm labor cannot be stopped, fetal mortality is increased primarily due to immature lungs and respiratory distress syndrome (RDS), decreased fat stores, and poor organ function, as well as increased risk of trauma during birth. Maternal stress is increased and treatments used to stop preterm labor may place the mother at risk for adverse reactions. Additional risk factors for preterm labor include non-white race, abdominal trauma, cervical incompetence, cervical dilation of 1 cm at 32 weeks, bleeding after 12 weeks, uterine abnormality, stress, prolonged standing, inadequate weight gain, clotting disorders, and pregnancy within 6 to 9 months of previous pregnancy.

SIGNS AND SYMPTOMS

- Uterine contractions: 4 in 20 minutes or 8 in an hour at 20 to 37 weeks.
- Cervical changes with dilation of >1 cm or effacement of 80% or greater at 20 to 37 weeks. Cervical shortening (less than 25 mm before term) is abnormal.

TEST RESULTS

- Fetal fibronectin (fFN), obtained by cervical swab, that is positive at 22 to 37 weeks gestation is highly predictive of preterm labor.
- Blood glucose (may indicate uncontrolled diabetes).
- Thyroid hormones may be elevated indicating thyrotoxicosis.
- Laboratory studies: Complete blood count (CBC), C-reactive protein, vaginal cultures, and urine culture to detect infections.
- Ultrasound may reveal short cervical length and fetal status.

TREATMENTS

- Bed rest in side lying position to maintain uterine blood flow.
- IV infusion for maternal hydration.
- **Tocolysis** (use of medications to arrest labor) includes the use of drugs such as β-adrenergic agonists/β-mimetics, most commonly magnesium

sulfate and terbutaline sulfate (Brethine), to contain uterine contractions and delay birth. These drugs also cause suppression of other maternal muscles and can result in side effects, including pulmonary edema.

- Fetal sedation and hypotonia may also result from administration of tocolytics but should resolve within 2 days after birth.
- Calcium channel blockers, such as nifedipine (Procardia), could be effective in arresting preterm labor.
- Prostaglandin synthesis inhibitors (PSIs) such as indomethacin (Indocin) may also be used; however, the side effects are severe, making this a less common treatment.

NURSING INTERVENTIONS

- Note mothers with risk factors for preterm birth.
- Monitor at-risk woman for uterine activity and teach her the signs of preterm labor, self-check methods to detect contractions, and the use of home uterine activity telemetry.
- Maintain regular contact with the at-risk woman.

Patient Education

- Teach the at-risk woman the signs of preterm labor:
  - Painful or painless uterine contractions every 10 minutes or less
  - Mild uterine cramps low in the abdomen
  - Abdominal cramping alone or accompanied by diarrhea
  - Continuous or intermittent sensations of pelvic pressure like the baby is descending
  - Membrane rupture
  - Continuous or occasional low, dull backache
  - Vaginal discharge that increases in amount, changes to pink tint, or becomes clear and watery
- Teach the woman to take measures to prevent preterm labor:
  - Rest up to 3 times daily lying on the left side.
  - Avoid lifting heavy objects.
  - Avoid overexertion.
  - Decrease or stop sexual intercourse, if needed, to decrease contractions.
  - Empty bladder every 2 hours to minimize stimulation.
  - Drink 2 to 3 quarts of water daily.
  - Avoid caffeine.
  - Minimize stress by focusing on each day and not trying to resolve all concerns at once.
- Teach the woman that if frequent contractions (every 10 minutes or less) are noted for an hour or other signs are present for an hour, or if clear vaginal fluid is noted, she should call her physician or midwife and arrange for an examination.

HEMORRHAGIC CONDITIONS

PLACENTA PREVIA

What Went Wrong?

In placenta previa the placenta is implanted in the lower portion of the uterus instead of the upper portion. The implantation over or near the cervical os presents the danger that as the lower uterus contracts and dilates in preparation for birth the placental villi are ripped from the uterine wall, creating open sinuses that will bleed into the space. The cause of placenta previa is unknown, but women who have given birth by cesarean section, women who are black or of other minority races, women with factors like multi parity (number of pregnancies in which fetus reached viability), and high **gravidity** (number of pregnancies), mothers of advanced age, women who have had prior miscarriage or induced abortion, cigarette smokers, and women giving birth to a male fetus are at higher risk for the condition. The condition can present in one of several forms depending on the degree to which the os is covered. The greater the degree to which the os is covered, the more severe the tearing and bleeding and the greater the danger to the fetus and mother. The uterus may present with (1) low implantation, without os covering; (2) partial placenta previa; or (3) complete placenta previa (see Fig. 9.1).

🔑 Signs and Symptoms

- ◑ Fetal heart rate: abnormal fetal heart rate 8 (i,e, bradycardia or variable deceleration: persistent, severe or late).
- ◑ Amniotic fluid may reveal meconium staining.
- ◑ Painless, bright red vaginal bleeding (may begin as scant and progress to profuse).

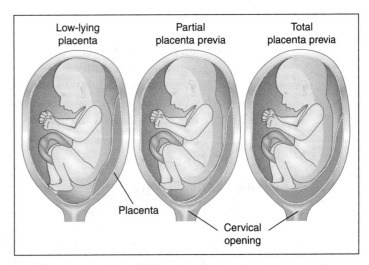

Figure 9.1 • Placenta previa at different cervical os/opening coverings.

Nurse Alert Do not perform a vaginal examination on an expectant mother with vaginal bleeding until placenta previa has been ruled out.

Test Results

- Transabdominal ultrasound reveals the placenta in a low portion of uterus.
- Hemoglobin and hematocrit may be decreased if bleeding has occurred.
- Rh factor and urinalysis may be performed to detect other possible complications.

Treatments

- If bleeding from placenta previa occurs before 37 weeks gestation, measures are taken to delay birth until at least 37 weeks for enhanced fetal maturity.
  - Monitor closely, bed rest (strict if bleeding is noted), and take vital signs every 4 hours.
  - Maintain IV fluids and type and cross-match 2+ units of blood and keep on hand.
  - Deliver at 37 to 38 weeks if fetal lungs are mature.
- If bleeding from placenta previa occurs after 37 weeks:
  - In low implantation or minimal placenta previa with head presenting down in pelvis, if scant to no bleeding is noted and fetal status is stable, a vaginal birth may be induced.
  - If partial or complete placenta previa is noted or continued bleeding is noted with minimal placenta previa, birth by cesarean is performed.

Nursing Interventions

- Monitor mother and fetus closely for signs of distress.
- Assist the woman in maintaining bed rest. Ambulation to the bathroom is allowed if no bleeding is noted.
- Monitor for bleeding.
- Note pain presence or level.
- Monitor uterine contractility.
- Use an external fetal monitor to evaluate fetal heart rate.
- Provide IV fluids as ordered.
- Infuse blood as indicated and ordered.

ABRUPTIO PLACENTA

What Went Wrong?

Abruptio placenta is the premature separation of the placenta from the uterine wall (see Fig. 9.2). The severe hemorrhage that results is the primary cause of death of the fetus and danger to the mother. Occurrence is usually after 20 weeks gestation, most often in the last trimester.

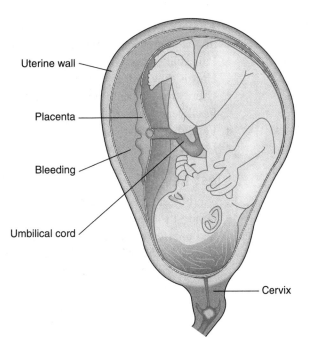

Uterine wall

Placenta

Bleeding

Umbilical cord

Cervix

Figure 9.2 • Abruptio placenta.

There are three types of abruptio placenta:

- ☽ Marginal/marginal sinus rupture: With placental separation at the edges with blood flowing between fetal membranes and the uterine wall to exit vaginally.
- ☽ Central: With placental separation in the center area, trapping blood between the placenta and the uterine wall. Blood does not exit vaginally and thus is hidden.
- ☽ Complete: With massive bleeding due to total separation of the placenta from the uterine wall.

The cause of abruptio placenta is unknown; however, risk factors for the condition include trauma to the abdomen (such as from a fall or car accident), advanced maternal age, history of high parity, cigarette smoking, maternal hypertension, rapid uterine emptying as occurs with hydramnios or multiple birth pregnancy, cocaine abuse, uterine fibroids or malformation, placental abnormalities, prior abruption, inherited thrombophilia, or preterm premature rupture of the membranes (PPROM).

🔑 Signs and Symptoms (will vary based on degree of separation)

- ☽ Sudden and ferocious onset.
- ☽ Tender, hard abdomen.
- ☽ Bleeding may be visible or concealed.
- ☽ Dark red venous blood.

- Anemia.
- Shock symptoms if blood loss is severe.
- Pain that is regular, severe, and localized to the uterine area.
- Uterus that is firm and hard to touch during contractions.
- Uterus may be enlarged or irregularly shaped.
- Fetal heart tones may be absent or present.
- Fetal distress may be evident.
- Fetal engagement may be noted.

Test Results

Abruptio placenta may be graded according to the symptoms presented:
- Grade 1 (40% of cases): Mild separation with minimal vaginal bleeding and unaffected fetal heart rate pattern and maternal blood pressure.
- Grade 2 (45% of cases): Partial separation with moderate bleeding and uterine irritability. Elevated maternal pulse and compromised fetal heart rate are noted.
- Grade 3 (15% of cases): Significant or complete separation of placenta with maternal shock noted and painful uterine contractions. Commonly causes fetal death.
- Hemoglobin and hematocrit decreased due to bleeding.
- Coagulation factors decreased.
- Disseminated intravascular coagulation (DIC) may occur (discussed in the next section).
- Ultrasound reveals location of placenta and absence of placenta previa.

Treatments

- Blood products to replace loss.
- Maintain hematocrit above 30%.
- Administer corticosteroid to facilitate fetal lung maturity.
- Administer immunoglobulin to women who are Rh-negative.
- Fluid volume replacement with IV fluids to keep urine output at 30 cc per hour or more.
- Deliver the fetus through vaginal delivery (if term) or cesarean delivery if fetal distress or other complications are noted.

Safety Alert **If DIC is present, cesarean delivery is contraindicated.**

Nursing Interventions

- Palpate for uterine tone and presence of tenderness.
- Monitor for bleeding, and note the rate, amount, and color.
- Monitor fetal heart rate pattern for signs of distress.
- Monitor maternal vital signs.
- Assess maternal respiratory and cardiac sounds.

- ◑ Monitor maternal skin color, turgor, and capillary refill.
- ◑ Monitor level of consciousness for signs of decreased circulation.
- ◑ Monitor urinary output.
- ◑ Monitor intake closely and adjust to maintain adequate urine output.
- ◑ Provide emotional support to the mother and family facing the crisis.

DISSEMINATED INTRAVASCULAR COAGULATION

🔑 What Went Wrong?

Disseminated intravascular coagulation (DIC) is a disorder of the blood clotting that is acquired as a result of excessive trauma as well as in many of the complications of pregnancy (such as abruptio placenta or retained products of conception after an abortion). In normal blood clotting a balance is maintained between the hemostatic (clotting) system and the fibrinolytic (dissolving) system. In DIC an imbalance occurs between clotting activity and fibrinolysis. Extreme clotting occurs in small areas of the circulatory system, decreasing the availability of clotting factors such as platelets and fibrin for the general circulation, leading to increased coagulation and a bleeding defect at the same time.

🔑 Signs and Symptoms

- ◑ Oozing of blood or uncontrolled bleeding may be noted from puncture sites from injections or IV therapy.
- ◑ Ecchymoses and petechiae form on the skin.
- ◑ Distal extremities (toes and fingers) may appear pale, cyanotic, or mottled and may be cold to the touch because small blood vessels are congested with coagulated blood, blocking circulation to the extremities.
- ◑ Neurologic or renal dysfunction may occur from occlusion of vessels supplying the brain and kidneys.

🔑 Test Results

- ◑ Platelet levels are decreased (thrombocytopenia): The level depends on the ability of and speed with which the bone marrow replaces platelets.
- ◑ Elevated fibrin split products.
- ◑ Extremely low serum fibrinogen levels (less than 100 mg/100 mL).
- ◑ Large-appearing platelets on blood smear, possibly fragmented (from passing through meshes of collecting fibrin).
- ◑ Prolonged prothrombin and partial thromboplastin times.

🔑 Treatments

- ◑ The first step is to resolve the initial insult, for example, deliver the infant and remove the abruptio placenta.
- ◑ Intravenous heparin is administered to interfere with the excessive coagulation.
- ◑ A blood transfusion may be needed to correct blood loss.

Nurse Alert **If ordered, the blood transfusion may need to be delayed until after heparin has been administered so that the new blood factors are not lost in the abnormal coagulation process.**

- Fresh-frozen plasma, platelets, or fibrinogen may be administered to promote clotting factors.
- Blood coagulation studies should return to normal range with adequate therapy; however, tissue damage occurs secondary to blocked blood vessels, for example, renal or brain cell damage, and permanent injury may result.

Nursing Interventions

- Assist as needed in the resolution of the underlying problem (see abruptio placenta, for example).
- Administer heparin and monitor clotting and bleeding activity.
- Explain the use of heparin in DIC to the mother and family, making certain to explain that bleeding will not be increased because clotting factors will be made available to promote clotting.

HYPERTENSIVE DISORDERS

PREGNANCY-INDUCED HYPERTENSION (PIH)

Conditions in pregnancy that result in hypertensive crisis (systolic blood pressure [BP] above 140 mm Hg and diastolic BP above 90 mm Hg) may range from mild to severe. Hypertension could also be measured as an increase of 30 mm Hg above pre-pregnancy systolic BP or 15 mm Hg above pre-pregnancy diastolic BP. These conditions include gestational hypertension, mild to severe preeclampsia, eclampsia, and the hemolysis, elevated liver enzymes, and low platelets (HELLP) syndrome. When not treated quickly, several associated conditions have been noted: maternal and fetal death, hepatic rupture, placental abruption, acute renal failure, or preterm birth.

What Went Wrong?

The contributing factors for the occurrence of PIH may be multifactorial and a specific cause has not been singled out. Possible changes during pregnancy, such as the lowered peripheral vascular resistance of early pregnancy that resolves after week 20 due to shifts in hormones, may be over-corrected, resulting in hypertension. Conditions involved in PIH may occur singularly or in combination:

- Gestational hypertension (GH): After week 20 of pregnancy the woman develops hypertension without proteinuria or edema. The hypertension resolves within 6 weeks after birth.
- Mild preeclampsia is the onset of GH in combination with 1+ to 2+ proteinuria and a weight gain of 4.4 pounds (2 kg) per week in the last two trimesters. Slight edema of the face or upper extremities is also noted.

- Severe preeclampsia is present when BP reaches or exceeds 160/100 mm Hg or higher, with 3+ to 4+ proteinuria, oliguria, cerebral or visual disturbances such as headache or blurred vision, serum creatinine above 1.2 mg/dL, hyperreflexia (ankle clonus may be noted), pulmonary or cardiac problems, thrombocytopenia, severe peripheral edema, hepatic dysfunction, and right upper quadrant and epigastric pain.
- Eclampsia includes severe preeclampsia symptoms in addition to seizures or coma. Warning signs of the onset of eclampsia include hyperreflexia, extreme epigastric pain, headache, and hemoconcentrations.
- **HELLP syndrome** is a form of gestational hypertension with severe preeclampsia with hepatic dysfunction in addition to coexisting hematologic conditions.

Signs and Symptoms

- Symptoms may vary based on the level of PIH being experienced and the organs being affected. Maternal vasospasm and poor circulation and nutrition delivery to the fetus can result in a low birth weight and premature infant.
- Hypertension of various levels will be noted.
- Protein in the urine ranging from 1+ to 4+.
- Neurologic symptoms such as visual blurring, headache, and hyperreflexia extending to coma may be noted.
- Liver dysfunction may occur.
- Epigastric or upper right quadrant pain may be reported and noted.
- Hemolysis—blood cell death—causes anemia and jaundice.
- Elevated Liver enzymes.
- Low Platelet count (<100,000/mm^3) or **thrombocytopenia** is noted with accompanying elevation in bleeding and clotting time, petechiae, bleeding gums, and disseminated intravascular coagulation (DIC).
- Nausea and vomiting and epigastric pain are noted.

Test Results

- Urine test may reveal proteinuria.
- 24-hour urine collection for creatinine clearance and protein.
- Elevated Liver enzymes (elevated alanine aminotransferase [ALT] or elevated aspartate transaminase [AST]).
- Complete blood count may reveal anemia (low hemoglobin and hematocrit) secondary to hemolysis.
- Abnormal clotting studies.
- Chemistry profile may reveal elevated creatinine and abnormal electrolytes due to impaired renal function.
- Nonstress test with biophysical profile.
- Serial ultrasounds and contraction stress test to determine fetus' status.
- Doppler blood flow evaluation to determine fetal and maternal status.

Treatments

Administer magnesium sulfate before or after PIH onset to depress vascular and neurologic activity, lowering blood pressure and preventing or stopping seizures.

Drug Alert **Signs of magnesium toxicity include absence of deep tendon reflexes, urine output below 30 cc per hour, respiratory depression (<12/min) and decreased level of consciousness.**

- **Administer antihypertensive medications.**
- **Low sodium diet.**
- **Bed rest in side-lying position.**
- **Fluid intake of 64 ounces daily (unless prohibited by renal failure).**

Nursing Interventions

Monitor pregnant women with risk factors for PIH closely for signs of onset, particularly those with age extremes (< 20 or > 40 years of age) or prior history of PIH.

- Maintain quiet environment with dim lighting to minimize stimulation of seizure activity.
- Keep airway open should seizure occur.
- Maintain bed rest, in side-lying position.
- Provide quiet activity and diversions.
- Enforce seizure precautions: Keep side rails up with padding as indicated, use padded tongue blade or keep oral airway at bed side.
- Observe client closely for seizure if she complains of epigastric pain (possibly related to vascular engorgement of the liver).
- Provide a diet that is low in caffeine and sodium.
- Teach the client to avoid alcohol intake.

Patient Education

Educate the client and family that at the onset of magnesium treatment sensations of flushing, feeling hot, and sleepiness may be noted.

- During magnesium infusion: Monitor vital signs, deep tendon reflexes, level of consciousness, visual acuity, report of headache, urinary output, epigastric pain, uterine contractions, and fetal status (activity and fetal heart rate).

 Nurse Alert **Monitor for signs of magnesium toxicity and if present discontinue drip, administer calcium gluconate as an antidote (should be standing order from physician), and have respirator and code cart available in case of arrest.**

 Safety Alert **Magnesium may cause sedation in the infant, and hypermagnesemia may also be noted in the newborn infant.**

ROUTINE CHECKUP

1. The nurse would expect to provide care for what condition if the expectant mother exhibited slight anemia; painless, bright red bleeding; and a soft, relaxed uterus?
   a. Hyperemesis gravidarum
   b. Placenta previa
   c. Abruptio placenta
   d. Ectopic pregnancy

Answer:

2. If an expectant woman is exhibiting hypertension, headache, decreased level of consciousness, proteinuria at 4+ level, and hyperreflexia with intermittent seizures, the nurse should note the woman is showing signs of what condition?
   a. Mild preeclampsia
   b. Gestational hypertension
   c. HELLP
   d. Eclampsia

Answer:

3. If a woman with PIH is on magnesium therapy and the nurse notes the urine output is 15 cc per hour and respirations are 8, the nurse should take what action?

Answer:

GESTATIONAL DIABETES

◢ WHAT WENT WRONG?

Gestational diabetes occurs when glucose intolerance is noted initially during pregnancy. The symptoms may resolve within weeks after delivery; however, in half of women diabetes mellitus develops within 5 years after delivery. With gestational diabetes the fetus is placed at higher risk for spontaneous abortion, exposure to maternal infections, hydramnios, ketoacidosis, hypoglycemia from maternal treatment of diabetes with insulin, skipped meals, increased exercise, or hyperglycemia with **macrosomia** (excessive fetal growth).

◢ SIGNS AND SYMPTOMS

- Maternal reports of intense or unusually frequent hunger or thirst (due to hyperglycemia).
- Urinary frequency.

- ◑ Blurred vision.
- ◑ Excess weight gain.
- ◑ Complications may be noted:
  - Hydramnios (increased volume of amniotic fluid).
  - Preeclampsia/eclampsia may be noted more frequently with gestational diabetes.
  - Ketoacidosis with possible coma and death of the fetus and mother.

TEST RESULTS

- ◑ Urinalysis reveals glycosuria and possibly acetonuria.
- ◑ 1-hour glucose tolerance test at 24 to 28 weeks indicates elevated glucose.
- ◑ 3-hour glucose tolerance test after fast reveals elevated glucose levels.
- ◑ Early pregnancy may show decreased blood glucose due to increased tissue responsiveness to insulin, while in late pregnancy tissue resistance to insulin may result in high blood glucose levels.

TREATMENTS

- ◑ Dietary management for pregnancy and diabetes control:
  - Increase calories to 300 kcal/day with 40%–45% coming from complex carbohydrates, 15%–20% from protein, and 35%–40% from fats.
  - Six meals (3 meals and 3 snacks) are preferable to prevent glucose fluctuation, with the night snack having a protein and a carbohydrate to prevent hypoglycemia in the night.
- ◑ Tight management of blood glucose with insulin is required:
  - Use lower doses in the first trimester due to increased tissue sensitivity and insulin antagonist human placental lactogen (hPL) levels.
  - Use higher doses in the last trimester as hPL levels are high with placental maturity and insulin is less effective.
  - High doses of insulin may be needed during labor to balance glucose.
  - A lower insulin dose may be needed with delivery of placenta and low hPL levels.
  - Insulin may not be needed during the postpartum period.
- ◑ Close monitoring of fetal development with anticipation of large-for-gestational-age child and accompanying complications if glucose is not well controlled.

NURSING INTERVENTIONS

Monitor timing carefully during glucose testing:

- ◑ 1-hour tolerance test (50 g oral glucose load followed by serum glucose analysis 1 hour later).

○ 3-hour tolerance test after overnight fast with no smoking or caffeine within 12 hours of test; glucose level drawn at 1, 2, and 3 hours after ingestion of 100-g glucose load.
○ Monitor blood glucose.
○ Monitor fetus.

Patient Education

○ Teach client and family the signs of:
  • Hypoglycemia (weakness; headache; nervousness; hunger; blurred vision; pale, moist skin; shallow respirations; rapid pulse; tingling extremities)
  • Hyperglycemia (thirst, increased urination, abdominal pain, nausea and vomiting, flushed skin, fruity [acetone] breath)
○ Discuss diet therapy and exercise for control of diabetes.
○ Educate the client on insulin administration techniques.
○ Administer insulin as ordered.

Nurse Alert **Avoid oral hypoglycemic agents, which are contraindicated in pregnancy because they cause birth defects.**

• **Instruct the mother to monitor fetal kicks and record the kick count.**
• **Discuss the possibility that adult-onset diabetes may follow gestational diabetes so follow-up monitoring is needed by the mother.**

CONCLUSION

Complications of pregnancy can occur at any stage, beginning with fertilization and through birth. The nurse has a role in determining the presence of a pregnancy complication at as early a point as possible to promote early intervention, if possible, to minimize fetal or maternal injury, or early termination of a non-viable pregnancy to minimize damage to the female reproductive system that may result in infertility. Key points addressed in this chapter include the following:

○ Fertilization of the egg does not guarantee a viable pregnancy, and growth of the fertilized egg in the fallopian tube can endanger the female if the tube ruptures and bleeding and shock result.
○ The nurse should support the mother and father/family in grief with a tubal pregnancy as with the loss of any pregnancy.
○ Hyperemesis gravidarum presents a risk to the pregnant female due to the loss of fluids, electrolytes, and nutrients with vomiting, and presents a risk to the fetus for intrauterine growth restriction and possible preterm and low weight birth.

○ Premature rupture of membranes presents a risk to the mother for infection and to the fetus for premature birth, prolapsed or compressed cord, or infection due to exposure to organisms.

○ Digital examinations are avoided with premature rupture of membranes to reduce exposure to pathogens.

○ Pregnancy is prolonged as long as possible if the fetus is less than 37 weeks gestation when membranes rupture, with maternal bed rest and hospitalization if indicated.

○ Preterm labor is treated with medication to stop labor (tocolytics) and decreased activity or bed rest.

○ Placental implantation near the cervical os (placenta previa) can increase the risk of placental tearing during birth, resulting in bleeding and decreased fetal oxygenation and hypoxia; cesarean birth is done in partial or complete placenta previa.

○ If vaginal bleeding is noted, do *not* perform a vaginal examination until placenta previa has been ruled out.

○ Fetal lungs are tested for maturity and delivery is delayed, if possible, until the lungs are mature (37 to 38 weeks).

○ Abruptio placenta is an acute situation requiring fetal delivery by the vaginal route if term or cesarean delivery if fetal distress is present and no DIC is present.

○ DIC can occur as a result of trauma or complications of pregnancy such as abruptio placenta.

○ Treatment for DIC involves heparin, an anticoagulant, which will release clotting factors from small vasculature and make those clotting factors available to promote clotting.

○ Preeclampsia and eclampsia, and gestational hypertension can increase the risk of maternal and fetal death or injury. The causes appear to be multifactorial so anticipation is not guaranteed, and early detection of symptoms is key in early treatment and control.

○ Management of magnesium sulfate requires monitoring closely for toxicity represented by excessive suppression of reflexes and respiratory depression.

○ Gestational diabetes presents a danger to the mother and fetus if blood glucose is not well controlled. The fetus can grow excessively from exposure to high glucose levels and, as a large-for-gestational-age newborn, will be at risk for hypoglycemia and other complications.

○ Early diagnosis of gestational diabetes promotes early management and a decreased impact on the fetus.

FINAL CHECKUP

1. **Which symptoms would suggest that a pregnant female may have an ectopic pregnancy?**
   a. An elevated serum hCG level
   b. An empty womb by ultrasound
   c. An elevated progesterone level
   d. No report of fetal activity by the 3rd week

2. **A woman diagnosed with hyperemesis gravidarum may be administered what medication?**
   a. Methotrexate
   b. Meperidine
   c. Metoclopramide
   d. Metraplasma

3. **What statement is accurate regarding premature rupture of membranes?**
   a. Digital examination should be performed every 2 hours to assess membrane status.
   b. Speculum examination reveals a vaginal fluid that tests positive by nitrazine paper test.
   c. Corticosteroids are given to restore membrane stability and repair rupture.
   d. If fetal lungs are mature and signs of infection are noted, a cesarean delivery is performed.

4. **The nurse should prepare for what treatment of the woman in preterm labor?**
   a. Oxytocin
   b. Brethine
   c. Thyroxine
   d. Glycogen

5. **Which symptom indicates the onset of premature labor?**
   a. Nausea
   b. Urinary frequency
   c. Abdominal cramping
   d. Difficulty breathing

6. **Which mother should the nurse watch most closely for placenta previa?**
   a. Mrs. Parker, who is a 22-year-old woman of European race
   b. Mrs. Barfield, age 28, who is a nullipara
   c. Miss Dennis, who is having a female child
   d. Mrs. Taylor, a 40-year-old in her third pregnancy

7. **Mrs. Daily has been diagnosed with complete placenta previa and is having continued vaginal bleeding with a 38-week fetus. What nursing care would be appropriate?**
   a. Prepare Mrs. Daily for vaginal birth.
   b. Insert an IV into Mrs. Daily for induction of labor.
   c. Ambulate Mrs. Daily to the bathroom to empty her bladder.
   d. Perform preoperative teaching for cesarean delivery.

8. **What treatment may be required for a woman with abruptio placenta?**
   a. Delivery of the fetus through vaginal delivery if fetal distress is noted
   b. Delivery of the fetus by cesarean birth if DIC is present
   c. Administration of immunoglobulin to decrease placental rupture
   d. Administration of corticosteroids to promote fetal lung maturity

9. **What assessment finding would indicate the presence of DIC?**
   a. Platelet count is increased.
   b. Fibrinogen levels are very low.
   c. Extremities are flushed red.
   d. Prothrombin time is short.

10. **A low-sodium diet, fluid intake of 64 ounces per day, and dim lights may be implemented for what condition?**
   a. Hypoglycemia
   b. Preeclampsia
   c. Gestational diabetes
   d. Hydramnios

ANSWERS

Routine Checkup
   1. b
   2. d
   3. Discontinue the infusion and administer calcium gluconate per standing order.

Final Checkup

1. b	2. c	3. b	4. b	5. c
6. d	7. d	8. d	9. b	10. b

CHAPTER 10

Labor and Delivery

Objectives

At the end of this chapter, the student will be able to:

1. Discuss theories that explain the initiation and progression of labor.

2. Discuss the signs and symptoms of labor and its progressive stages.

3. Discuss treatment regimens and nursing interventions associated with each stage of labor and delivery.

4. Discuss assessments and diagnostic findings related to complications of labor and delivery.

5. Discuss the care for a woman and newborn secondary to complications experienced in labor and delivery.

KEY TERMS

Attitude	Lightening
Breech presentation	Non-reassuring
Cephalic presentation	Passage
Decelerations	Passenger
Dilation	Position
Effacement	Powers
Engagement	Reassuring
Episiotomy	Ripening
Leopold's maneuvers	Station
Lie	Transition

OVERVIEW

Although most times the labor and delivery process is a long-awaited end to a pregnancy, it can be painful for the expectant mother and anxiety provoking for the mother and family. The onset and progress of labor has been explained through various theories or hypotheses:

- Prostaglandin connection: While the presence of prostaglandins appears to stimulate labor and the blocking of prostaglandins seems to stop premature labor, the exact mechanism of prostaglandins in the labor process is unknown. Prostaglandins are associated with rising levels of estrogen and oxytocin, platelet activating factor, and endothelin-1.
- Progesterone withdrawal hypothesis: Since progesterone plays a part in relaxing the uterus, withdrawal of this calming effect through biochemical changes that occur when birth is near allows estrogen to dominate and stimulate uterine contractions.
- Corticotropin-releasing hormone (CRH) levels increase as the end of pregnancy gets nearer (and has been noted in preterm labor). CRH stimulates the production of prostaglandins (F and E). The increased prostaglandin levels contribute to the stimulation of uterine contractions.

THE LABOR PROCESS

Each component of the labor process has a distinct role:

1. **Passenger** includes the fetus and the placenta. The fetal head size, lie, presentation, position, and attitude will impact the passing of the fetus through the birth canal. Since the placenta must also pass through the birth canal, it is also a passenger.

◑ **Fetal head size** is measured by the anterior-posterior diameters of the skull as well as the transverse diameters (biparietal and bitemporal diameters). As the head is flexed or extended different diameters (occipitofrontal, submentobregmatic, suboccipitobregmatic, or occipitomental) present to the maternal pelvis.

◑ **Lie** is the cephalocaudal relationship of the fetal longitudinal axis (spinal column) to the maternal spinal column. The fetal lie can be parallel or longitudinal to the maternal spine (vertical up and down/in alignment with the maternal spine) or transverse (side to side/horizontal at right angle to the maternal spine).

◑ **Fetal attitude** is the way fetal body parts relate to one another, particularly degree of flexion and extension. The usual attitude is moderate head flexion with arms flexed to the chest, and legs flexed to the abdomen. This results in the smallest part of the head presenting to the maternal pelvis.

◑ **Presentation** is the fetal lie and the body part that approaches the birth canal first. The fetal presentation can be head first (cephalic), hips first (breech), or shoulder first.

1. **Cephalic presentation** is the most common and is described based on the area of the head presenting.

    a. **Vertex** is the most frequent presentation with the fetal neck flexed to the chest and the suboccipitobregmatic diameter presenting to the mother's pelvis.

    b. **Military** presentation occurs when the fetal neck is straight and the top of the head (occipitofrontal diameter) presents to the mother's pelvis.

    c. **Brow** presentation occurs when the fetal neck is extended, partially allowing the upper face (occipitomental diameter) to present first to the maternal pelvis.

    d. **Face** presentation occurs when the fetal neck is hyperextended and the face (submentobregmatic diameter) presents to the maternal pelvis.

2. **Breech presentation** occurs when the fetal hips and feet present toward the maternal pelvis.

    a. Complete breech is noted when both the knees and hips of the fetus are flexed and the hips and feet of the fetus present to the maternal pelvis.

    b. Frank breech is noted when the hips of the fetus are flexed and the knees are extended, resulting in the hips presenting to the maternal pelvis.

    c. Footling breech occurs when the fetal hips and the legs are extended and one or both of the fetal feet present to the maternal pelvis.

3. **Shoulder presentation** occurs when the fetus is in transverse lie and the shoulder, arm, abdomen, back, or side presents to the maternal pelvis.

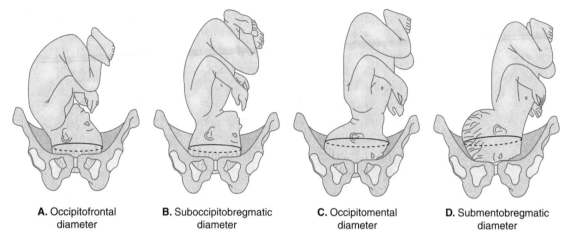

A. Occipitofrontal
diameter

B. Suboccipitobregmatic
diameter

C. Occipitomental
diameter

D. Submentobregmatic
diameter

Figure 10.1 • Multiple categories of presentation.

Recording of the fetal position is done by indicating the relationship of the presenting fetal part to the maternal pelvis:

- ☽ The first letter represents the side of the maternal pelvis: Right (R) or left (L).
- ☽ The second letter represents the presenting part of the fetus: Head/occiput (O), hips/sacrum (S), face or chin/mentum (M), or acromion process of the scapula (A or Sc).
- ☽ The third letter represents the aspect of the maternal pelvis: Anterior (A), posterior (P), or transverse (T). For example, ROP = right occiput posterior (see Fig. 10.1).

Fetal position is determined by the practitioner through use of **Leopold's maneuvers**, a series of abdominal palpations to assess the fetal presenting part, fetal attitude, lie, descent, and best location for auscultation of fetal heart tone on the maternal abdomen. The Leopold's maneuvers are performed with the woman on her back with her knees bent and her feet on the bed to relax the abdominal muscles.

 Nurse Alert **Perform maneuvers between contractions and instruct the woman to empty her bladder prior to beginning the maneuvers to promote comfort and reduce disruption of palpation due to a full bladder.**

Maneuvers are as follows:

First: Facing the mother, the nurse should palpate the upper abdomen with both hands noting the mobility, shape, and consistency of the palpated part to determine if the fetus' head or buttocks are at the fundus (top of the abdomen). The head will feel round and solid and will move separately from the larger trunk, while the buttocks are soft with bony knobs (hip bones) and they move with the trunk (Fig. 10.2A).

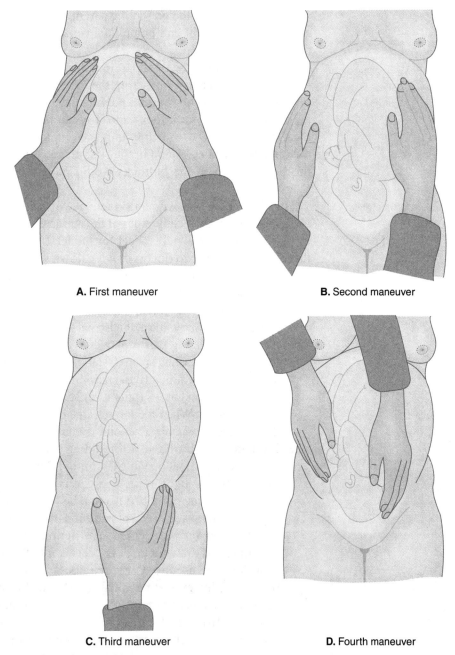

A. First maneuver

B. Second maneuver

C. Third maneuver

D. Fourth maneuver

Figure 10.2 • Leopold maneuvers.

Second: Locate the fetal back by using palms to palpate the abdomen with gentle deep pressure. Hold the right hand stable while exploring the right side of the uterus with the left hand. Repeat the step holding the left hand stable and exploring the left side of the uterus. The fetal back is smooth and firm and should lead from the presenting part noted in the first maneuver. The fetal extremities feel small and bumpy/uneven and should be opposite the back (Fig. 10.2B).

Third: Determine the fetal part that lies just above the pelvic outlet (presenting part) by gently squeezing the lower abdomen just above the symphysis pubis with the thumb and fingers. Note if the part feels like the hard head or the soft buttocks and if it can be gently pushed forward and back (not engaged) or is firmly in place (engaged). The findings should be the opposite of those found in the first maneuver (if the head was noted in the first maneuver, the buttocks would be noted in the third maneuver) (Fig. 10.2C).

Fourth: Facing the woman's feet, place hands on the maternal lower abdomen and gently feel the sides of the uterus while sliding both hands down toward the symphysis pubis. Feel for the fetal brow by noting the side with the highest resistance to fingers moving downward. Note if the brow is on the side opposite the back (the fetal head is flexed) or on the same side as the back (the fetal head is extended) (Fig. 10.2D).

1. **Engagement:** The fetal descent into the pelvis is measured in centimeters using an imaginary line at the ischial spines as the landmark and noting if the fetal presenting part is above/superior to the line (minus station), at the level of the ischial spine (0 station), or below/inferior to the line (plus station). At −5 (minus five) station the fetus is just entering the pelvis (pelvic inlet) and at +5 (plus five) station the fetus is ready to be born (pelvic outlet). When the largest area of the presenting fetal part passes through the pelvic inlet (station 0), **engagement** has occurred (Fig. 10.3).

2. **Passage:** The birth canal, including the pelvis, pelvic floor, cervix, vagina, and vaginal opening (introitus). The fetus must be able to move into the pelvis and through the cervix and vagina; therefore, the size and shape of the bony pelvis must be large enough to allow fetal passage. The adequacy of the preparation of the cervix for delivery is evaluated based on the degree of dilation (opening) and effacement (thinning and drawing up of the cervix into the uterine wall). A Bishop score may be used to assess readiness for delivery. Using a scale of 0–3, five elements are evaluated—cervical dilation, cervical effacement, cervical position (midline, anterior, or posterior), cervical consistency (firm, medium, soft) and station of presenting part. If the score is 9 or higher for first deliveries/nulliparas, or 5 or more for multiparas, the cervix is determined to be suitable for labor and induction can be performed if indicated.

   Cervical ripening may be promoted with medication (prostaglandin gel/Cytotec, Prepidil) or mechanical measures (balloon catheters, dilators or sponges with magnesium sulfate inserted into cervix, or laminaria tents with desiccated seaweed) to promote induction of labor.

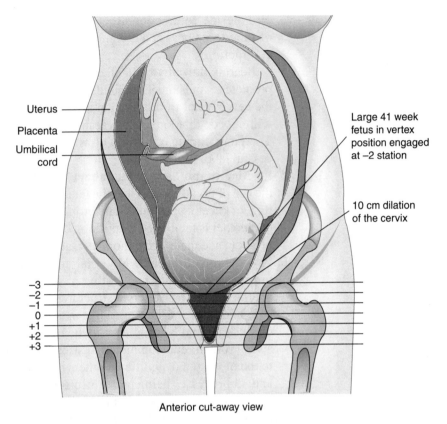

Uterus

Placenta

Umbilical
cord

Large 41 week
fetus in vertex
position engaged
at −2 station

10 cm dilation
of the cervix

−3
−2
−1
0
+1
+2
+3

Anterior cut-away view

Figure 10.3 • Fetal descent stations (Birth Presentation).

The nurse should monitor for urinary retention, rupture of membranes, uterine pain, contractions, vaginal bleeding, or fetal distress during the procedure. The number of dilators or sponges used should be documented.

3. **Powers** include uterine contractions and maternal bearing down and pushing to expel the fetus. The strength of uterine contractions, along with the amniotic fluid between the fetal head and maternal cervix during the descent, plays a major role in placing pressure on the cervical opening, contributing to uterine dilation and effacement. Maternal ability to push and bear down is critical to the vaginal delivery of the newborn without external assistance.

Contractions are evaluated based on the **frequency**, the time from the beginning of one contraction to the beginning of the next contraction; the **duration**, the time between the beginning and the end of a contraction; the **intensity**, the strength (mild, moderate, or strong) of a uterine contraction at its peak; and the **resting tone**, relaxation of the uterus between the end of one contraction and start of a new contraction.

Bearing down by the mother, once the cervix is dilated and effaced, promotes expulsion of the child. However, bearing down and pushing on the cervix prior to full dilation and effacement can cause swelling that will impede dilation and can result in trauma and tearing of the cervix. Therefore, timing of bearing down by the mother is important to a successful labor process.

4. **Position of mother during labor:** The maternal position can promote the use of gravity to assist in the fetal descent. An upright, squatting, sitting, or kneeling position could promote fetal descent. The well-being of the mother is facilitated by position changes during the labor period that promote adequate circulation, rest, and comfort.

5. **Psychological impact:** Maternal anxiety and stress can impede the progression of labor by creating physiological changes that counteract the relaxation of pelvic structures as needed to promote fetal passage and delivery. This tension can distract the mother from focusing on pushing and bearing down when appropriate. The nurse can play a vital role in reducing maternal stress through providing information to the mother and significant others regarding the progression of labor and all processes being performed for and with the mother, providing direction related to comfort measures, and listening to and addressing any concerns as quickly and calmly as possible. Calm partners and calm practitioners impact the psychological status of the laboring woman.

 ROUTINE CHECKUP 1

1. The fetal position and head size are considered under what factor that impacts labor and delivery?
   a. Passage
   b. Passenger
   c. Power
   d. Position of the mother

Answer:

2. What initials would the nurse use to describe a fetus that is presenting with the hips facing the anterior portion of the right side of the maternal pelvis?

Answer:

INITIAL (PREMONITORY) CHANGES PRECEDING LABOR

- Backache: Constant, dull low backache caused by pelvic muscle relaxation. If the fetus is positioned in a posterior presentation back pain may be more intense.
- Contractions progress from Braxton-Hicks (irregular intermittent false labor that do not change in frequency or duration or discomfort level despite activity; localized in abdominal area, no cervical dilation or effacement associated) to true labor (regular contractions with increasing frequency, intensity, and duration radiating from the back to the abdomen; progressive cervical dilation and effacement are associated).
- Lightening: Descent of the fetal head into the maternal pelvis about 2 weeks before the onset of labor. Often accompanied by increased urinary frequency due to pressure on bladder.
- Cervical changes: Ripening occurs with a softening of the cervix to allow stretching and thinning.
- Bloody show: Vaginal drainage of brown-red blood-tinged mucus due to the release of the cervical mucous plug when the cervix dilates.
- Rupture of membranes releasing 500 to 1200 cc of yellow, clear, watery fluid with no foul odor, confirmed with nitrazine paper turning blue indicating alkalinity of amniotic fluid (not acidic urine).
- Weight loss of 0.5 to 1.4 kg (1 to 3 pounds).
- Gastrointestinal (GI) changes (indigestion, diarrhea, nausea, and vomiting) may occur.
- Sudden high-energy surge.

LABOR PROCESS

The fetus proceeds through the birth canal for vaginal delivery through a process of:

- Engagement, when the largest (biparietal) diameter of the head of the fetus moves to station 0.
- Descent, when the presenting part moves through the pelvis from negative station to 0 and progresses to positive station.
- Flexion, when the fetal head flexes to bring the chin close to the chest and presents the smallest diameter of the head to the maternal pelvis for passage through the cervix and out of the vagina for birth.

STAGES OF LABOR

The woman and child undergo specific changes during each stage of labor proceeding to vaginal delivery. The stages of labor vary in duration depending upon this being a first delivery for the woman (primigravida), or the second or higher delivery (multigravida).

○ **Stage 1** begins with the onset of labor and has 3 phases:

a. Latent phase

    i. Cervix 0 cm (begins) to 3 cm dilation (ends).

    ii. Contractions are irregular and progress from regular to mild to moderate, 5 to 30 minutes apart, 30 to 45 seconds duration.

    iii. Partial cervical dilation and effacement.

    iv. Spontaneous rupture of membranes (SROM) or artificial rupture of membranes (AROM).

    v. Mother is talkative and eager.

b. Active phase: Stage 1 ends 8 to 20 hours (primigravida) or 2 to 14 hours (multigravida) after reaching this phase.

    i. Cervix 4 cm (begins) to 7 cm dilation (ends).

    ii. Contractions are regular, moderate to strong, 3 to 5 minutes apart, 40 to 70 seconds duration.

    iii. Cervix dilated 7 cm with rapid effacement.

    iv. Fetal descent begins.

    v. Mother becomes more anxious and restless as contractions intensify; feelings of helplessness may be reported.

c. Transition phase: Ends when dilation is complete at 10 cm.

    i. Cervix 8 to 10 cm dilation

    ii. Contractions regular, strong to very strong, 2 to 3 minutes apart, 45 to 90 seconds duration.

    iii. Mother is tired, irritable, and restless, and feels helpless and unable to handle labor (this is the hardest phase of labor).

    iv. Nausea and vomiting and a sensation of needing to have a bowel movement may be noted.

    v. Urge to push noted.

    vi. Bloody show increases as amniotic fluid escapes.

○ **Stage 2:** Duration of 30 minutes to 3 hours for primigravidas, and 5 to 30 minutes for multigravidas; begins with full dilation and ends with delivery of the placenta.

- Pushing ends in delivery of the fetus (or if complications occur and alternate delivery is required). In most vaginal deliveries, the fetal head position moves through flexion, internal rotation, extension, restitution and external rotation, then expulsion from the maternal body:

- **Flexion:** During vaginal delivery the fetal head pushes against the cervix, pelvic floor, or pelvic wall, and the head flexes against the chest to place the smallest diameter for passage through the pelvis.

- **Internal rotation:** The fetal occiput rotates laterally and anterior while moving in a twisting motion past the ischial spines through the pelvis.

- **Extension:** The fetal occiput exits under the maternal symphysis pubis then veers anteriorly. The head is "born" as it exits the vagina by extension of the chin up and away from the fetal chest.
- **Restitution and external rotation:** After the head exits the vagina it rotates into alignment with the fetal body and makes a 1/4 turn as the shoulder exits under the maternal symphysis pubis and exits the vagina.
- **Expulsion:** With the head and shoulders out of the vagina, the remaining newborn body flexes toward the maternal symphysis pubis and is born.

◐ **Stage 3:** Duration of 5 to 30 minutes primigravidas/multigravidas; begins with delivery of the newborn and ends with delivery of the placenta.

- Placenta separates and is expelled—one of two surfaces emerges first:
  ○ Schultze: Shiny fetal side of placenta presents first.
  ○ Duncan: Dull maternal side of placenta presents first.

◐ **Stage 4:** Duration of 1 to 4 hours primigravidas/multigravidas; begins with delivery of the placenta and ends when mother's vital signs stabilize.

- Vital signs stable
- Lochia scant progressing to moderate rubra

FETAL ASSESSMENT DURING LABOR AND DELIVERY

The stress of labor can impact the fetus in positive and negative ways. The process of labor and delivery works to prepare the fetus for birth and the initial breath that will launch the newborn into extrauterine life. Fetal assessment is vital during the labor and delivery period to determine fetal tolerance of the labor and general well-being. Assessments performed and desired findings include:

◐ Fetal heart rate (FHR) monitoring:

- Performed by auscultatation with fetoscope or intermittent Doppler monitor held at maternal abdominal area where fetal back lies (lower quadrants in cephalic presentation, upper in breech presentation, near maternal umbilicus if transverse lie).
- As the fetus descends into the pelvis the FHR descends and moves toward the maternal midline.
- 🔑 Normal FHR is 110 to 160 beats per minute (bpm), with slight **variability** (change in FHR over a brief period of seconds to minutes). Normally, a short increase in FHR (**acceleration**) occurs with fetal stimulation (increased oxygen demand) or uterine contractions due to brief hypoxia from compression on the cord (reduced fetal oxygen supply). This compensatory mechanism indicates a healthy responsive

fetal autonomic nervous system. Decreased variability may indicate fetal sleep (increases with stimulation) or more serious fetal problems such as sedation with drugs that depress the nervous system, fetus <32 weeks with immature neurologic control of heart rate, neurologic damage, fetal anomalies of the heart, fetal dysrhythmias, or hypoxia with acidosis. Absence of variability is a serious warning sign.

- Count FHR for at least 30 seconds (multiply by 2 for rate/minute). Listen for a full minute after a contraction to detect anomalies and assess whether rate is abnormal (outside range), or if deceleration or irregularity is noted.
- Initiate continuous electronic monitoring (CEM) if anomaly is noted.
  - History of previous stillbirth at 38 weeks or more.
  - Complication of pregnancy suspected or diagnosed (preeclampsia, placenta previa, or other).
  - Induction of labor (with Pitocin or other measures).
  - In cases of preterm labor.
  - Decreased movement of the fetus.
  - Fetal status shows signs of distress (nonreassuring).
  - Meconium staining of amniotic fluid (indicates fetus is stressed by a problem and evacuated bowels in response).
  - Trial of labor after prior cesarean delivery.
  - Maternal fever.
  - Placental complications (inadequate oxygenation of fetus)
- Compare maternal heart rate to FHR to ensure that the monitor is tracking the fetus's and not the mother's heart rate.
- Electronic FHR monitoring can be external using a transducer on the mother's abdomen, or internal using a probe attached to the fetal presenting part.
  - Mother must be confined to bed.
  - Membranes must have ruptured.
  - Cervix must be dilated 2 cm or greater.
  - Presenting fetal part must be against the cervix.

 Nurse Alert **The presenting part must be distinguished to avoid placement of the probe on genitalia, or over an eye or fontanel.**

- Obtain a baseline FHR for at least 2 minutes, avoiding periodic or episodic shifts resulting in change in rate >25 bpm. Baseline rate, variability, and timing of changes in FHR in relation to contractions are noted during FHR assessment.
- Assess FHR when membranes rupture, after ambulation, after administration of drugs, after a procedure (i.e., vaginal examination, enema, etc.), or with any abnormal uterine activity.

- **Decelerations** are decreases in FHR from the baseline that occur early, late, or at variable times during a uterine contraction.
  - **Early deceleration** occurs at the onset or early stage of a contraction secondary to compression of the head by uterine constriction, with the peak depression of rate as the contraction peaks and return to baseline rate after the contraction. Rate remains within FHR range. This fetal response is deemed **reassuring** (normal).
  - **Late deceleration** occurs well after a contraction moves toward or passes peak due to decreased flow of blood and oxygen to the fetus often secondary to compromised placenta blood flow with maternal hypotension (due to epidural or oxytocin) or other condition such as maternal hypertension, diabetes, vascular disorder, or placental abruption. Immediate delivery or cesarean delivery may be indicated. Early and late decelerations occur gradually over 30 seconds or more.
  - **Variable decelerations** occur at different times during a contraction secondary to obstructed blood flow from the fetus to the placenta with a resulting fetal hypertension that stimulates the aortic arch and carotid baroreceptors to slow FHR. The deceleration is abrupt/sudden (<30 seconds).
  - Decelerations can occur in an episodic fashion without relationship to contractions or periodically in relation to contractions (they are considered repetitive if occurring with half or more of the contractions). Prolonged decelerations last for more than 2 minutes but less than 10 minutes.
  - If decreased or absent variability is noted with late or variable decelerations, tracing is viewed as **nonreassuring** (troubling) and acute treatment and continued monitoring are indicated.
- Wandering baseline FHR tracings reveal an unsteady baseline with no variability and may indicate the following:
  - Congenital defects.
  - Metabolic acidosis.
  - Requires oxygen to be administered.
  - The baby is to be delivered as quickly as possible.
- Fetal tachycardia (rate above 160 bpm) or marked tachycardia (>180 bpm) may indicate complications:
  - Fetal hypoxia
  - Maternal dehydration
  - Maternal fever
  - Maternal intake of drugs that stimulate the heart (such as atropine or terbutaline)
  - Intrauterine infection and amnionitis

- ○ Fetal anemia
- ○ Maternal hyperthyroidism
- ○ Tachydysrhythmias (rare)
- Fetal bradycardia can be harmless or may indicate distress (particularly in combination with decreased variability and late decelerations). Bradycardia may be caused by the following:
  - ○ Late fetal hypoxia
  - ○ Maternal hypotension
  - ○ Umbilical cord compression (vagal stimulation slows pulse)
  - ○ Fetal complete heart block or congenital heart block
  - ○ Uterine hyperstimulation
  - ○ Uterine rupture
  - ○ Maternal hypothermia
  - ○ Abruptio placenta
  - ○ Vagal stimulation in the second stage

 ROUTINE CHECKUP 2

1. The nurse would instruct the mother to pack her hospital bag and prepare for delivery within the next 2 weeks if the mother reported what information?
   a. Passing blood clot and 5 pads a day of bright red blood
   b. Feeling dizzy and tired with a 4-pound weight gain this month
   c. Having to void often but having less trouble breathing than last week
   d. Feeling no movement or activity from the fetus for the past 2 weeks

   Answer:

2. The fetal head is at the maternal pelvis with the largest diameter fully pressing into the opening of the maternal pelvis. The fetal head is in the process of _____ and is at ____ station.

   Answer:

MATERNAL AND FAMILY CARE

The laboring mother and family move through various processes and emotions as labor proceeds through to delivery. At each stage the nursing care is focused on assessment for complications, providing comfort and minimizing anxiety through communication and anticipation, and addressing the needs of the laboring mother, the fetus, and the family.

STAGE 1

◑ Monitor vital signs every 4 hours until the membranes rupture then increase monitoring to every 1 to 2 hours. If fever (>37.5°C[99.6°F]) is present, monitor temperature every hour. Notify physician/midwife if blood pressure is over 135/85 mm Hg or systolic is below 100 mm Hg or pulse is outside the range of 60 to 100 bpm, and perform vital sign assessment more frequently (avoid doing vital signs during periods of painful contractions).

◑ Assess maternal pain level (on a scale of 1–10). Provide comfort measures to reduce discomfort as much as possible—reposition, massage, etc.

◑ Palpate uterine contractions for frequency, duration, and intensity every 1/2 hour, or every 15 minutes for high-risk women. Uterine relaxation should be noted between contractions.

◑ Nursing care includes the following:
  • Responding to any questions or verbalized needs
  • Reinforcing prenatal teaching and preparations for labor and delivery, including breathing techniques
  • Assisting the mother to a position of comfort and changing the position as desired.

Nurse Alert **If the fetus demonstrates late decelerations, position the mother on the left side to improve fetal circulation.**

  • Provide oral care and comfort measures if vomiting is noted; provide clear fluids as desired and tolerated.

Fetal Assessment

◑ Record fetal heart rate (FHR) every 30 minutes, or every 15 minutes for high-risk pregnancies. Monitor rate and regularity, and note the **variability** (fluctuations in FHR per minute), and deceleration (early or late). The desired range is 110 to 160 beats per minute. A fetal heart monitor should be attached to the laboring mother to allow continuous monitoring if FHR is not within the 110 to 160 range, or late or variable decelerations are noted.

Latent Phase
Maternal Care

◑ Continue monitoring vital signs every hour if normal, and more frequently (every 15–30 minutes) if findings are outside of normal range as stated above.

◑ Offer the mother ice chips or a mouth swab (or a lollipop) to relieve dry mouth from labor breathing.

- ◐ Clear liquids as desired (stop fluids within 2 hours of planned cesarean delivery, and stop solid food within 6 hours of an elective surgery).
- ◐ Continue emotional support of mother and family.

Fetal Care

- ◐ Continue to monitor FHR and report findings outside expected variability or if late or variable deceleration is noted.

Active Phase

This phase is characterized by more frequent contractions (every 2–5 minutes) that are of greater intensity and duration (40–60 seconds).

- ◐ Assist the woman to a position of comfort, which is often in a bed or a reclining chair if desired.
- ◐ Palpate contractions every 15 to 30 minutes and note if uterine relaxation occurs between contractions.
- ◐ Perform vaginal examination to assess cervical dilation (usually 5–7 cm) and effacement, fetal station, and fetal position, and determine if membranes have ruptured.

Nurse Alert **Limit exams to avoid introduction of bacteria into the vaginal tract.**

- ◐ To maintain maternal comfort, change the perineal pad frequently due to soiling with vaginal discharge and increased amounts of bloody show.
- ◐ Assess pain level, provide comfort measures, and assist with medical relief of pain, if indicated.
- ◐ Encourage the woman to void since a full bladder can slow fetal descent. Catheterize if she is unable to void.
- ◐ Note the amount and other characteristics (color, odor, and consistency) of the fluid when the membranes rupture. Fluid should be clear without odor. Assist in the rupture of membranes if spontaneous rupture does not occur.

Fetal Care

- ◐ Monitor FHR every 30 minutes (15 if high risk).
- ◐ Note the presence of meconium (green-brown fluid) in the amniotic fluid when rupture occurs as this may indicate of fetal distress.
- ◐ Monitor for signs of complications (such as decreased variability or drop in FHR, which may indicate prolapsed cord or placenta previa). Interventions include the following:
  - • Monitor FHR continuously.
  - • Position the mother in knees to chest or Trendelenburg position.
  - • Administer oxygen per standing orders.
  - • Notify physician or midwife.
  - • Prepare for cesarean delivery if ordered.

Transition

This phase is characterized by contractions every 11/2 to 2 minutes that are strong and are 60 to 90 seconds in duration.

Maternal Care

- Assess for dilation (8–10 cm) and effacement (100%).
- Palpate contractions every 15 minutes, along with vital sign assessment.
- Frequent sterile vaginal examination to note rapid changes in preparation for delivery.
- Provide comfort for the woman, who may experience nausea or vomiting, shaking, and high anxiety (along with anticipation) during intense contractions.
- Provide or encourage the support person to provide a backrub or other physical contact, if desired. Encourage the woman to breathe slowly between contractions and try to rest, when able; during contractions encourage panting and pursed-lip breathing to avoid hyperventilation and prevent pushing until cervix is fully dilated.
- Evaluate coping of mother and family. Answer questions clearly and repeat as needed. Explain that fatigue is expected and encourage rest.
- Provide analgesics if ordered and monitor maternal and fetal response. Provide a quiet room to promote rest between contractions.
- Offer ice chips and apply lubricant to dry lips.
- Position for comfort when pushing is allowed. Support legs during pushing.

Fetal Care

- Monitor FHR every 30 minutes (every 15 minutes in high-risk pregnancy)
- Provide support measures and notifications if rate falls outside parameters. Attach monitor to allow for frequent FHR assessment as indicated.

STAGE 2

This stage begins with complete dilation and effacement of the cervix and ends with birth of the newborn.

Maternal Care

- Assess for dilation (10 cm) and effacement (100%).
- Palpate every contraction and pushing effort of the woman, along with vital sign assessment.

- Assess for increased bloody show as a sign of impending delivery.
- Monitor FHR continuously every 10 minutes, or more often if problems are noted, and following birth.
- Watch for perineal lacerations, particularly at the time the head is born. Note depth of laceration:
    - First degree: Tear extends through the skin and superficial structures.
    - Second degree: Tear extends through the skin, muscles, and into the perineum.
    - Third degree: Tear extends through the skin, muscles, perineum, and the muscle of the anal sphincter.
    - Fourth degree: Tear extends through the skin, muscles, anal sphincter, and the rectal wall.

To avoid extension of the laceration into muscle and the anal area a surgical incision (episiotomy) is performed to control/prevent tearing.

- Reposition the woman for the most effective position to support pushing efforts.
- Assist the support person in encouraging and coaching the woman through pushing efforts with bearing down during contraction.
- If fecal matter is released during labor, clean perineal area.
- Encourage rest between contractions and deep breathing.
- Encourage the woman by reporting progress, including when fetal head is visible, has descended out, and as remaining body parts emerge.
- Confirm the gender of the newborn and explain that baby will be cleaned and the cord cut before the baby is brought to the mother. If desired, the father/labor partner may cut the cord.
- Provide contact between the newborn and the mother and family to promote early bonding. If indicated, contact with the mother's breast is made to initiate the newborn's suck reflex and stimulate contractions to promote expulsion of the placenta.

Fetal Care

- Throughout labor and delivery monitor FHR for signs of distress.
- Upon delivery of the fetal head, suction the nose and mouth to remove secretions and encourage breathing; observe the nature of the cry, if present.
- Immediately after birth of all body parts observe the newborn's color, respirations, and muscle tone.
- Clean the fluid from the newborn's body, and after the cord is cut wrap the newborn in a blanket and present the newborn to the mother and family.
- Perform initial assessment (Apgar) of the newborn, then send the newborn to the nursery.

STAGE 3

This stage involves the delivery of the placenta, usually within 30 minutes of the newborn's birth.

- Continue monitoring of mother's vital signs every 15 minutes.
- Evaluate fundus for contraction and note signs of placental separation:
  - Sudden dark blood flow from vagina.
  - Umbilical cord length extends as placenta descends.
  - Vagina fills with placental mass.
- Encourage the mother to push when placental separation is evident.
- Promote maternal-infant contact to stimulate the release of oxytocin, which will stimulate uterine contraction and the release of the placenta.
- Administer oxytocin as ordered to promote uterine contractility to prevent hemorrhage after the placenta is expelled. Uterine massage may be performed to stimulate contraction.
- Cleanse the perineal area with saline or warm water and apply a perineal pad (apply an ice pack if desired, particularly if episiotomy is performed).
- Return the mother to bed for rest (or if bed was converted for birth restore it to the resting position).

STAGE 4

(See Chap. 11: Postpartum Care.)

MATERNAL COMFORT AND SUPPORT

Maternal comfort is critical during the labor and delivery process. As indicated in Chapter 8 on childbirth preparation, there are many choices in pain control ranging from distraction, physical contact, and relaxation, to spinal blocks. A combination of pharmacologic and non-pharmacologic measures can reduce the total amount of medication needed and the negative effects on the mother and child.

- Perform pain assessment with maternal vital sign assessment.
- Assist the mother into a position that provides maximum comfort and change positions as often as needed.
- Change the pads under the mother, and linen if needed, and cleanse the perineum to remove draining fluids and promote comfort.
- Encourage support person(s) to assist the mother as needed with distraction techniques, ice chips for dry mouth, and other measures that provide physical comfort such as effleurage or back rubs.
- Monitor the effect of medications and spinal blocks, if applied.
- Maintain hydration by offering fluids as often as allowed to prevent hypotension from spinal blocks.

POSITIONING FOR VAGINAL DELIVERY

A woman may assume varied positions during the labor and delivery process. The use of gravity is beneficial to promote fetal descent and each position has benefits and disadvantages. Ultimately, maternal choice in addition to position effectiveness will determine the position used for child birth.

- Recumbent position is often assumed using a birthing bed or a bed with head elevated and legs in stirrups. The nurse should monitor for pressure from the uterus on the maternal diaphragm and tilt the mother to the left side if indicated to relieve pressure on the major blood vessels. Cushions may be applied between the stirrups and legs to reduce pressure.
- Lateral Sims' position: Lying on the left side with the upper leg elevated decreases pressure on major blood vessels and may relax perineal structures. Maternal visibility of the delivery may be reduced.
- Squatting: Increases the size of the pelvic outlet to promote fetal passage and may shorten the second stage of labor. Mother may have difficulty maintaining this position so assistance may be needed.
- Sitting in a bed or in a birthing stool/chair allows gravity to assist with the birth with minimal pressure on major blood vessels. Back support should be provided by the support person or nurse.
- Positioned on hands and knees increases perineal relaxation and promotes fetal descent and rotation. In addition, greater access to fetus is provided. The mother will have a limited view of the birth and may become fatigued more easily. Support pillows should be provided. Adjust the bed and mirrors, if present, to allow maximum view by the mother.

USE OF DELIVERY ASSISTANCE MEASURES

If labor does not spontaneously progress to expulsion of the fetus, measures may be needed to increase the passageway, or push or pull the fetus through the vaginal passage.

- **Labor induction** may be needed.
  - If spontaneous labor does not occur prior to 42 weeks.
  - If labor is prolonged due to inadequate uterine contractions.
  - If membranes are ruptured, leaving the mother and fetus at risk for infection.
  - If there are maternal complications such as Rh incompatibility, diabetes, eclampsia, or pulmonary disease.
  - If there is fetal death.
  - Prostaglandins may be applied to the cervix, oxytocin (Pitocin) may be given intravenously, amniotomy (rupture of membranes) may be performed, or nipple stimulation may be done to trigger oxytocin release.
  - Nursing assessment includes the following: Cervical readiness, FHR, and uterine contractions

Nurse Alert **Report signs of hyperstimulation.**

- Assess baseline FHR prior to amniotomy and monitor throughout and after procedure. Note color, consistency, amount, and odor of amniotic fluid and document along with time of procedure.
- Assess that fetus is engaged in birth canal at 0 or positive station prior to initiation of oxytocin. Obtain a Bishop score prior to beginning the drug. Monitor contraction frequency, duration, and intensity, along with FHR every 15 minutes and with dosage changes, and maternal vital signs every 30 minutes and with each dose titration. Monitor maternal intake and output.
- Regulate oxytocin as ordered to obtain a contraction frequency of every 2 to 3 minutes and a duration of 60 to 90 seconds with an intensity of 40 to 90 mm Hg per intrauterine pressure catheter (IUPC); uterine resting tone is 10 to 15 mm Hg, and FHR remains within range (110–160 bpm).
- Stop oxytocin if contraction frequency occurs less than every 2 minutes, duration exceeds 90 seconds, intensity exceeds 90 mm Hg, uterine resting tone is above 20 mm Hg between contractions, no uterine relaxation is noted between contractions, or FHR is abnormal in rate, variability, or decelerations (late, variable, or prolonged).
- If uterine hyperstimulation is noted contact the primary care provider, position the woman on her left side, provide IV fluids as ordered, apply oxygen, administer tocolytic (terbutaline[Brethine]) to relax the uterus, and monitor FHR and uterine activity and record.

◖ An **episiotomy**, an incision to the vaginal opening to enlarge it during fetal passage, may be performed to prevent tearing of tissue during delivery (controversial).
- Indications for use include the need to shorten labor, permit forceps-assisted delivery, remove premature fetus with minimal fetal trauma, and assist the birth of a large (macrosomic) newborn.
- Median/midline incision (easier to repair and more effective) may be made or mediolateral episiotomy (greater blood loss) may be performed. Third-degree lacerations may occur with both; fourth-degree lacerations are associated with midline incisions. Local anesthetic is applied prior to the incision. Nursing care is noted in chapter 11: Postpartum Care.

◖ **Forceps or vacuum-assisted birth** may be performed if the mother is unable to push effectively or fetal distress is noted. Forceps may be needed if fetal rotation stops, or abnormal fetal presentation or breech delivery requires assistance delivering the fetal head (Fig. 10.4).
- **Nursing assessments include the following:**
  ◦ FHR prior to, during, and after the use of forceps (cord compression may cause decreased FHR requiring repositioning of forceps).
  ◦ Client should empty her bladder or be catheterized.

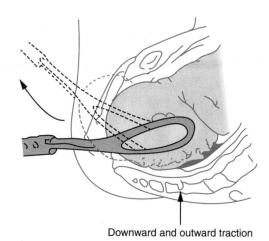

Downward and outward traction

FIGURE 10.4 • Forceps delivery.

○ Verify that membranes are ruptured and fetus is engaged in the pelvis.
○ Monitor the newborn for bruising after delivery.
○ Monitor the mother for vaginal or cervical laceration (hemorrhage even if uterus is contracted), urinary retention due to urethral or bladder trauma, or hematoma formation from blood vessel rupture.
○ Explain the procedure to the mother and support persons and reassure them that bruises and hematoma on the scalp, if present, will resolve.
○ Position in lithotomy or ordered position.
○ 🔊 Report to the newborn nursery and postpartum nurses that forceps or vacuum delivery was performed to promote continued monitoring.

THE CESAREAN DELIVERY

WHAT WENT WRONG?

A cesarean delivery is indicated when vaginal delivery is not safe due to problems with the maternal pelvis or vaginal passage that pose potential danger to the newborn or mother.

🔊 SIGNS AND SYMPTOMS

Assessments that may indicate that cesarean delivery is needed may include the following:

◐ Fetal position that is not occipital (head first) such as breech or acromion.
◐ Insufficient or compromised placental blood supply to the fetus such as might occur with placenta previs, abruptio placenta, or prolapsed cord.
◐ Difficulty in inducing labor when immediate delivery of the fetus is needed for medical reasons.

- Large fetal size (>9 lb or more).
- Possible maternal distress or potential injury secondary to a condition that may be worsened by the stress of labor, such as heart disease or eclampsia.
- Open sores from active genital herpes or human immunodeficiency virus (HIV) infection, both of which can be passed to the fetus during vaginal delivery.
- Multiple pregnancy: The direction and size of the incision depends on the position of the fetuses. In particular, cesarean delivery may be needed for multiple births involving:
    - Twins if one amniotic sac is shared (monoamniotic twins), due to the risk that the cords will get tangled
    - Multiple fetuses (three fetuses or more)
    - Known anomalies that would make vaginal delivery difficult, i.e., conjoined (Siamese) twins
- Poorly positioned, large, or multiple fetuses cause an overstretched uterus that cannot contract adequately during labor (uterine inertia), making labor long and difficult.

TEST RESULTS

- Ultrasound may reveal measurements of the maternal pelvis and fetus that indicate a risk for problems with fetal descent through the pelvis (cephalopelvic disproportion).
- FHR that indicates decreased or absent variability, late decelerations, or variable decelerations, indicating the need for emergency cesarean birth.
- Maternal or fetal distress with labor, indicating the need for emergency cesarean birth.
- Labor that fails to progress, indicating the need for unplanned cesarean birth.
- Cultures of the mother reveal infection that could pass to the fetus during vaginal delivery.

TREATMENTS

- Cesarean delivery may be planned such as when the maternal pelvis size is too small for a large fetus, resulting in a head-to-pelvis mismatch (cephalopelvic disproportion). Repeat cesarean may be needed if each pregnancy reveals this problem.
- Emergency cesarean delivery is indicated if labor fails to progress and maternal or fetal distress is noted and immediate birth is needed for maternal or fetal safety.
- The direction and size of the incision depends on the position of the fetus(es):
    - Transabdominal incision may be utilized.
    - Horizontal incision in the lower segment of the uterus is the most currently used.

◑ Labor may be allowed to attempt vaginal delivery on a later pregnancy even if a cesarean was done during a prior pregnancy.

◆ NURSING INTERVENTIONS

◑ Preoperative care involves the following:
  - Obtaining an informed consent from the mother
  - Assessing maternal vital signs and FHR; obtaining preoperative lab work and diagnostics as ordered
  - Assisting the mother and family and answering questions; assisting the support person if attending the birth, and explaining what to expect and how to support the mother
  - Restricting intake as ordered (nothing by mouth beginning at midnight prior to the surgery), and assessing the last meal if an emergency cesarean is ordered and notifying anesthesiology
  - Positioning the client supine in a lateral tilt to shift weight off the vena cava and aorta (using a wedge under the hip)
  - Teaching deep breathing and coughing exercises for use after delivery to promote airway clearance postoperatively
  - Inserting urinary catheter
  - Administering preoperative medications and preparing the surgical site as ordered
  - Inserting an intravenous line, if not already present

◑ Postoperative care is similar to care after abdominal surgery:
  - Monitor vital signs frequently (every 15 minutes, then 30 minutes, then hourly during the early postoperative period and decreasing to every 4 hours when the mother stabilizes).
  - Assess pain and provide pharmacologic and non-pharmacologic relief measures.
  - Monitor for and report complications of cesarean birth:
    ◦ Aspiration or other anesthesia-related complications
    ◦ Amniotic fluid pulmonary embolism
    ◦ Infection—wound, urinary tract
    ◦ Hemorrhage
    ◦ Thrombophlebitis (blood clots)
    ◦ Wound dehiscence
    ◦ Bladder or bowel injury
    ◦ Fetal injury due to surgery
    ◦ Premature fetal birth secondary to error in gestational age

 Nurse Alert **If vaginal delivery is attempted in a mother with a history of cesarean delivery, monitor for risk factors for uterine rupture during labor, such as having a vertical scar, three or more cesarean scars, triplets or more, or a very large fetus thought to weigh 9 to 10 lb or more.**

• See Chapter 11 on postpartum care for additional measures for maternal care after delivery, and Chapter 12 on newborn care for measures needed for the newborn.

CONCLUSION

◑ The onset and progress of labor has been explained through various theories/hypotheses including the following:
  • Prostaglandin connection with stimulation of labor.
  • Progesterone withdrawal hypothesis, indicating the lack of progesterone to relax the uterus results in uterine contractions.
  • Corticotropin-releasing hormone (CRH) levels increase and stimulate prostaglandins, which results in stimulation of uterine contractions.
◑ Labor involves a combination of factors that will impact the transition from first contraction to delivery. These factors include the passenger (fetus and placenta), passage (cervical dilation and effacement), powers (contractions and maternal bearing down), maternal position (gravity), and psychological impact.
◑ Leopold's maneuvers are a series of palpations used to identify fetal presenting part, fetal attitude, lie, and descent as well as fetal heart tone location.
◑ Initial/premonitory signs precede labor, including backache, Braxton-Hicks contractions, lightening, cervical changes, bloody show, rupture of membranes, weight loss, GI distress, or energy surge.
◑ During labor the fetal presenting part moves from a negative station to engagement at the pubis (station 0) to a positive station and then out for birth.
◑ The stages of labor include the following:
  • Stage 1: The onset of labor until full cervical dilation (10 cm) and effacement (100%) (**latent, active, and transitional phases**)
  • Stage 2: Full dilation through delivery of the fetus through head flexion, internal rotation, extension, restitution and external rotation, then expulsion
  • Stage 3: Delivery of the placenta—shiny Schultze fetal side or dull Duncan maternal side presenting first
  • Stage 4: Immediate postdelivery period until maternal vital signs stabilize
◑ Fetal assessment should reveal FHR between 110 and 160 bpm with variability and acceleration of FHR with activity. Bradycardia, tachycardia, absence of variability, or late or variable deceleration are indications of fetal distress.

FINAL CHECKUP

1. **What is a sign of maternal distress during labor?**
   a. Less intense and less frequent uterine contractions
   b. Uterine relaxation between 50-second contractions
   c. Heart rate of 90 to 100 beats per minute during labor
   d. Reports of needing to have a bowel movement

2. **Which change is theorized to stimulate the onset of labor?**
   a. Decreased prostaglandin production
   b. Elevated corticotropin-releasing hormone (CRH) levels
   c. Increased progesterone production
   d. Oxytocin, platelet activating factor, and estrogen withdrawal

3. **Patricia Nealy is admitted to the maternity wing for a scheduled cesarean delivery. Why would the nurse teach deep breathing exercises as part of the preoperative preparation?**
   a. To prevent mucus buildup in the alveoli of the lungs
   b. To avoid contraction of the muscles of the diaphragm
   c. To promote uterine involution during the surgery
   d. To stimulate pulmonary edema absorption

4. **If the nurse notes a fetal heart rate (FHR) of 90 during the active phase of labor what action would be appropriate?**
   a. Encourage the mother to relax and check again in 15 minutes.
   b. Assist the mother to stand up and walk around to stimulate the fetus.
   c. Apply oxygen per standing orders and notify the primary care provider.
   d. Continue the same schedule of monitoring of FHR and maternal vital signs.

5. **During the transition phase of labor what would the nurse expect to observe?**
   a. The mother is calm and in minimal discomfort.
   b. The fetal heart rate is minimally affected by the contractions.
   c. Support person(s) are coaching the mother in panting.
   d. Six to ten minutes are noted between contractions.

6. **What would be an appropriate nursing intervention for fetal care during labor?**
   a. Monitor FHR every 30 minutes for a high-risk pregnancy.
   b. Maintain the mother in a supine position to promote fetal circulation.
   c. Report findings of FHR above 110 and below 160 beats per minute.
   d. Administer oxygen to the mother if variability in FHR is reduced.

7. **Which sign should cause the greatest concern if noted by the nurse?**
   a. Maternal irritability during the transition phase of labor
   b. Amniotic fluid that is green-brown in color
   c. FHR that is variable and increased with contractions
   d. Contractions of 40-second duration in the active labor phase

8. **Which is an appropriate plan for vaginal examination during labor?**
   a. Assess for cervical dilation and effacement every 30 minutes when labor begins.
   b. Assess for cervical ripening every 30 minutes during the latent phase,
   c. Examine the mother during the peak of contraction to determine impact on the cervix.
   d. Perform frequent sterile vaginal examinations during the transition phase of labor.

9. **What factors indicate the need for an emergency cesarean delivery?**
   a. Failure of labor to progress
   b. Maternal cardiac distress
   c. Fetal distress
   d. All of the above
   e. b and c only

10. **Nursing care following a cesarean delivery would involve what measures?**
   a. Wound care to the episiotomy
   b. Monitoring for cervical ripening
   c. Encouraging deep breathing and coughing
   d. Infusing oxytocin to promote placental delivery

ANSWERS

Routine Checkup 1
   1. b
   2. RSA

Routine Checkup 2
   1. c
   2. engagement ... zero/0

Final Checkup

1. a	2. b	3. a	4. c	5. c
6. d	7. b	8. d	9. d	10. c

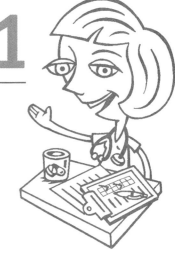

CHAPTER 11

Postpartum Care

Objectives

At the end of this chapter, the student will be able to:

1 Identify the priorities of maternal care given during the fourth stage of labor.

2 Describe the anatomic, physiologic, and psychological changes that occur during the postpartum period.

3 Identify characteristics of uterine involution and differentiate between the lochia flows.

4 Discuss interventions to prevent infection and excessive bleeding, promote normal bladder and bowel patterns, and care for the breasts of women who are breast-feeding or bottle-feeding.

5 Discuss discharge teaching and postpartum home care.

6 Identify causes, signs and symptoms, possible complications, and medical and nursing management of postpartum hemorrhage.

7 Discuss the causes of postpartum infection and summarize the assessment and care of women with postpartum infection.

8 Describe thromboembolic disorders, including incidence, etiology, clinical manifestations, and management.

9 Discuss postpartum emotional complications, including incidence, risk factors, signs and symptoms, and management.

KEY TERMS

After birth pains	Lochia alba
Diastasis recti	Lochia rubra
Disseminated intravascular	Lochia serosa
coagulation (DIC)	Mastitis
Embolism	Mood swings
Endometritis	Postpartum depression (PPD)
Engorgement	Postpartum hemorrhage
Fourth stage of labor	Puerperal infection
Hematoma	Puerperium
Hemorrhagic (hypovolemic)	Pulmonary embolism
shock	Subinvolution
Homans' sign	Thrombophlebitis
Involution	Thrombus
Lochia	Uterine atony

OVERVIEW

The postpartum period is generally considered to be the first 6 weeks after the birth of the infant and the return of the maternal reproductive organs to their normal nonpregnant state. This period is sometimes referred to as the fourth trimester of pregnancy, or **puerperium**. During the postpartum period the mother will experience a number of physiologic and psychosocial changes as the body returns to the pre-pregancy state. Pregnancy and childbirth are natural functions that most women recuperate from without complications. However, there are a number of physiologic and psychological complications that may occur during the postpartum period. The first part of this chapter focuses on anatomic, physiologic, and psychological changes that occur in the mother during the postpartum period. The second part of this chapter focuses on postpartum complications such as hemorrhage, subinvolution of the uterus, shock, infection, thromboembolic disorders, and psychological complications.

THE FOURTH STAGE OF LABOR

The first 1 to 2 hours after the birth of the baby is considered the **fourth stage of labor**. The fourth stage of labor is a crucial time for the mother and baby:
- ◗ They are both recovering from the physical process of birth.
- ◗ Maternal organs start the initial readjustment to the pre-pregnancy state and body system functions begin to stabilize.

◐ Nursing assessment is critical during this phase. All vital parameters such as pulse, respirations, O$_2$ saturation, blood pressure, lochia flow, level of consciousness, uterine firmness and position, motion and sensation (activity level), perineum, and color are assessed every 15 minutes for the first hour. Temperature is assessed during the initial observation and at the end of the first hour.

POST-ANESTHESIA RECOVERY

Women who give birth via cesarean or who had anesthesia require evaluation in the post-anesthesia recovery room or obstetrical recovery room.

◐ The required post-anesthesia recovery (PAR) score will be used to evaluate the mother's readiness for discharge from the area. Components of the PAR score include activity, respirations (respiratory status), blood pressure, level of consciousness, and color.

◐ The mother's activity, respirations, blood pressure, level of consciousness, and skin color and temperature are assessed every 15 minutes for the first 1 to 2 hours.

◐ The woman who has given birth by cesarean or who has received regional anesthesia for a vaginal birth requires special attention during the recovery period. The mother is discharged from the recovery room when she is stable.

◐ The transfer report will include information from the records of admission, birth record, and recovery.

• The report should include the following:
  ○ Name and age
  ○ Physician
  ○ Gravidity and parity
  ○ Anesthetic used; medications given
  ○ Duration of labor
  ○ Type of birth; any surgical repairs
  ○ Blood type, rubella status, and Rh status
  ○ Assessment of vital signs and summary of findings
  ○ Status of fundus, perineum, and bladder
  ○ Information regarding the baby's sex, weight, and preferred feeding method

PHYSIOLOGIC CHANGES OF THE REPRODUCTIVE SYSTEM

UTERINE INVOLUTION AND DESCENT OF THE UTERINE FUNDUS

Involution refers to the reduction in size of the uterus after birth, and its return to its pre-pregnant state. The involution process begins immediately after the delivery of the placenta when uterine muscle fibers contract:

- The uterine muscle contractions compress the blood vessels and control bleeding.
- Oxytocin is released from the pituitary gland to strengthen and coordinate the uterine contractions.
- To ensure that the uterus remains firm and well contracted during the first 1 to 2 hours postpartum, exogenous oxytocin (Pitocin) is generally administered intravenously or intramuscularly immediately after the expulsion of the placenta.
- It is crucial to monitor the mother closely during the first 1 to 2 hours postpartum to detect any signs of hemorrhage and prevent hypovolemic shock.

The uterus undergoes a rapid reduction in size and weight. At the beginning of the fourth stage of labor, the uterus is midline and can be palpated midway between the symphysis pubis and umbilicus:

- The uterus weighs approximately 2.2 pounds immediately after birth.
- Through the process of cell catabolism the size of individual cells in the uterus is reduced, causing a decrease in the size of the uterus.
- Within 12 hours after delivery, the fundus may be approximately 1 cm above the umbilicus and continues to descend approximately 1 cm or one fingerbreadth per day.
- During the first week the uterus decreases its weight by half, and by 2 weeks postpartum the uterus weighs approximately 12 ounces.
- The placenta site heals through a process of exfoliation, which leaves the uterine lining free of scar tissue.

The entire 6-week postpartum period is needed to complete uterine involution.

▲ UTERINE FUNDUS ASSESSMENT, OBSERVATIONS, AND INTERVENTIONS

- Explain the procedure.
- Ensure that the bladder is empty.
- Have the client assume a supine position with knees slightly flexed.
- Don gloves and apply a perineal pad in order to observe lochia as the fundus is massaged.
- Place one hand above the symphysis pubis to support the lower uterine segment during palpation or massage. With the dominant hand palpate the abdomen until the top of the fundus is located. Determine firmness.
- If the fundus is difficult to locate or soft, maintain the position of the hand above the pubis and use the dominant hand to massage the fundus with the flat surface of the fingers until firm.
- Note any lochia and any expelled clots.
- Document the consistency of the fundus (fundus firm, firm with massage, or boggy).
- Document the height of the uterus.

AFTERPAINS

Afterpains are cramping pains caused by intermittent uterine contractions. The pain is generally greater for multiparas versus first-time mothers due to the repeated stretching of the muscle fibers. The use of exogenous oxytocic medications and breast-feeding intensify the pain because they both increase uterine contractions. Assessments and required intervention may include the following:

- Assess pain using a standardized scale (facial grimaces or numeric).
- Administer analgesics as ordered.
- Position the patient in a prone position with a small pillow under the abdomen to help keep the uterus contracted, which aides in pain relief.

LOCHIA

Vaginal discharge during the puerperium consisting of blood, tissue, and mucus, commonly called **lochia**, initially is bright red and later changes to a pinkish red or reddish brown. It may contain small clots. In the first 1 to 2 hours post birth, the uterine discharge is similar to a heavy menstrual period. The redness of the lochia and the amount of lochia decrease throughout the postpartum period and generally ends 4 to 6 weeks postpartum. Lochia flow is scant in post-cesarean births. Lochia flow increases with breast-feeding and ambulation. Lochia flow is often heaviest when the mother gets out of bed due to the pooling of blood in the vagina during periods of rest. The nurse assesses lochia for quantity, type, and characteristics.

Nurse Alert **Not all postpartum vaginal bleeding is lochia; vaginal bleeding after birth may be caused by vaginal or cervical lacerations. Table 11.1 summarizes the characteristics of normal and abnormal uterine discharge.**

Recording the amount of lochia on the perineal pad by the hour is one method used for assessment (Fig. 11.1). Institutions differ on the agreement of terms for measuring amounts of uterine discharge so review the agency policies.

Type	Time Frame	Normal	Abnormal
TABLE 11.1 • Characteristics of Lochia			
Lochia rubra	1 to 3 days	Red vaginal flow consisting mostly of blood; small clots; fleshy odor	Foul odor; large clots; saturated perineal pad
Lochia serosa	4 to 10 days	Serous; pink or brownish, watery; decreased flow	Continuous or recurrent red color; excessive drainage; foul odor
Lochia alba	11 days to 6 weeks	Creamy white; light yellow; decreased amount	Recurrent lochia rubra; continuous lochia serosa; foul odor

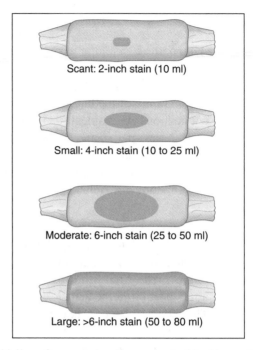

Figure 11.1 • Guidelines for assessing the amount of lochia on the perineal pad.

CERVIX

After birth the cervix is formless with an opening wide enough to insert the hand. The wide opening allows for manual examination of the uterus and manual extraction of the placenta if necessary. Within the first week postpartum the external os opening is approximately the width of a pencil.

VAGINA AND PERINEUM

The vagina usually appears stretched, edematous, and bruised, and the vaginal opening often gapes open when there is an increase in intra-abdominal pressure. By the third week postpartum the vaginal mucosa heals.

Postdelivery the perineum is edematous. The perineum may have torn during delivery or the mother may have a surgical incision (episiotomy) to the perineum. Although the tear or episiotomy is small, an incision in this area can cause a considerable amount of discomfort. Hemorrhoids may occur during pregnancy and during delivery.

NURSING INTERVENTION FOR RELIEF OF PERINEAL DISCOMFORT

- Use aseptic technique and don gloves for perineal care.
- Teach the appropriate technique for perineal care (wipe from front to back).

- ◐ Teach the mother how to perform a sitz bath.
- ◐ Instruct the mother on the use of topical anesthetics and astringent pads if ordered.
- ◐ Assess pain level and administer analgesics as needed.

✔ ROUTINE CHECKUP 1

1. What are the priorities for care during the fourth stage of labor?

Answer:

_____

_____

2. The process in which the uterus returns to a nonpregnant state after birth is known as

_____.

Answer:

3. What are the defining characteristics of lochia rubra, lochia serosa, and lochia alba?

Answer:

_____

_____

4. List interventions for the relief of perineal discomfort postdelivery.

Answer:

_____

_____

🕮 CARDIOVASCULAR SYSTEM

The cardiovascular system goes through tremendous changes during pregnancy (Table 11.2). During pregnancy, there is approximately a 40% to 50% increase in circulating blood volume (hypervolemia), which allows the mother to tolerate significant blood loss at birth without adverse effects. Many women lose at least 400 to 500 mL of blood during vaginal births and approximately twice as much during cesarean births.

During the first 72 hours after childbirth, there is a greater reduction of plasma volume than in the number of blood cells. This results in a rise in hematocrit and hemoglobin levels by the seventh day after the birth. There is no increased red blood cell (RBC) destruction during the puerperium, but any excess will disappear gradually in accordance with the life span of the RBC. The exact time at which RBC volume returns to pre-pregnancy values is not known, but it is within normal limits when measured 8 weeks after childbirth.

TABLE 11.2 • Cardiovascular System Changes	
Cardiac output	Initial ↑ in cardiac output post birth. The ↑ is caused by the following factors: ◐ ↑ blood flow back to the heart from the elimination of the placenta, which diverts 500 to 750 mL of blood flow into the maternal systemic circulation ◐ Rapid ↓ in the size of the uterus, which ↓ pressure on the vessels ◐ The movement of excess extracellular fluid into the vascular compartment
Plasma volume	Initial ↑ in plasma volume post birth. The body eliminates excess volume through the following mechanisms: ◐ Diuresis (increased excretion of urine), in which a daily urinary output can be as much as 3000 mL during the first 5 days (Blackburn, 2003)
Coagulation	Clotting factors are ↑ during pregnancy to reduce the risk of postpartum hemorrhage. The clotting factors remain ↑ for up to 4 weeks postpartum. This places the mother at ↑ risk for thrombus formation.
Blood values	◐ The hemoglobin and hematocrit levels are difficult to interpret during the first 3 days after birth due to the remobilization and rapid excretion of excess body fluids. The hemoglobin and hematocrit levels generally reach the pre-pregancy levels within 4 to 8 weeks postpartum. In the first 72 hours postpartum there is an ↑ in plasma loss that results in temporary hemoconcentration. Normal plasma values (30–45 mL/kg) return within 2 to 4 weeks postpartum. ◐ Leukocytosis occurs immediately post birth, with the white blood cell count increasing as high as $16,000/mm^3$. The white blood cell level returns to normal ($5000–10,000/mm^3$) within 10 days.

GASTROINTESTINAL SYSTEM

Digestion becomes active soon after childbirth. The mother is frequently thirsty and hungry after birth due to the tremendous amount of energy expended during the birthing process and the extended period without water or food. Clear liquids are given prior to solid foods. The diet can be advanced as tolerated. Constipation is commonly a problem during the postpartum period due to the following:

1. Decreased peristalsis caused by the remaining relaxing effects of progesterone
2. Stretched abdominal muscles, which make it difficult to bear down to expel stool
3. Soreness and swelling of the perineum and hemorrhoids
4. Fear of pain

If an episiotomy was performed, a stool softener or a laxative may be prescribed to avoid the discomfort of straining. A bowel movement is expected within 2 to 3 days after delivery. The mother is encouraged to increase fluid intake and regular ambulation daily.

URINARY SYSTEM

During pregnancy the bladder has increased capacity and decreased muscle tone. Also, during the delivery, the urethra, bladder, and tissue around the urinary meatus may become edematous and traumatized. Urination is also hindered by anesthetic drugs. The diminished awareness of the need to urinate may result in decreased sensitivity to fluid pressure, and the woman may not feel an urge to void. This is important to remember because the bladder fills rapidly as a result of intravenous fluids administered during labor and the diuresis process that follows birth. Urinary retention and over-distention of the bladder may lead to urinary tract infection and postpartum hemorrhage. With bladder distention, the uterus is displaced (often to one side, usually the right) and has a reduced ability to contract. When the uterus fails to contract, blood vessels are free to bleed. Therefore, it is important that the nurse monitor the woman for voiding and a distended bladder.

SIGNS AND SYMPTOMS OF A DISTENDED BLADDER

- Fundus is above the umbilicus.
- Fundus is displaced from the midline.
- Bulging of the bladder above the symphysis pubis.
- Frequent urination of less than 150 cc.
- Increases or excessive lochia.
- Tenderness over the bladder.

NURSING INTERVENTIONS

- To promote urination have the mother sit in the upright position.
- Run warm water over her hands.
- Pour water over the perineum to stimulate voiding. It is easy, noninvasive, and should be tried early on.
- The nurse may try oil of peppermint because it releases vapors that may relax the necessary muscles.
- Administer pain medication if the mother fears the urination process will be painful, which could interfere with her ability to void.
- Insertion of a catheter is invasive and should be the last intervention attempted.

MUSCULOSKELETAL SYSTEM

MUSCLES AND JOINTS

During the first few days post birth, many women experience muscle fatigue and ache. With the delivery of the placenta, the effect of progesterone on muscle tone is removed. Therefore, muscle tone begins to be restored throughout the body. The abdominal muscles, including the rectus abdominis muscles,

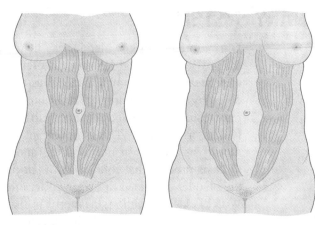

Figure 11.2 • Diastasis recti occurs with separation of the longitudinal muscles of the abdomen during pregnancy.

may be separated—**diastasis recti** (Fig. 11.2). Special exercises can strengthen the abdominal wall. Women need to be advised that with proper diet, exercise, and rest, abdominal muscle tone is usually regained more rapidly. Correct posture and good body mechanics are essential to help relieve low back pain. Encourage Kegel exercises to help the pubococcygeal muscle (muscle that aids bowel and bladder control) to regain normal function.

INTEGUMENTARY SYSTEM

Soon after childbirth the hormone levels begin to decrease and the skin gradually returns to the pre-pregnancy state. The melanocyte-stimulating hormone (MSH), estrogen, and progesterone levels, which cause hyperpigmentation during pregnancy, decrease rapidly after childbirth. Striae gravidarum (stretch marks), which develop on the abdomen, thighs, and breasts, gradually fade.

NEUROLOGICAL SYSTEM

Neurologic changes during the postpartum period result from a reversal of maternal adaptations to pregnancy and trauma from the birth process. The periodic numbness and tingling of fingers that trouble 5% of pregnant women usually disappear after the birth unless lifting and carrying the baby aggravates the condition. Postpartum headaches require careful assessment because they may result from a variety of conditions, including gestational hypertension, stress, and leakage of cerebrospinal fluid caused during placement of the needle for epidural or spinal anesthesia (Lowdermilk, Perry, Alden, Cashion, & Corbett, 2006).

ENDOCRINE SYSTEM

Estrogen and progesterone levels decrease after the expulsion of the placenta. If the mother is bottle-feeding, estrogen levels begin to rise to follicular levels approximately 2 to 3 weeks after delivery, which allows the return of menses. Pre-pregnancy levels of estrogen and progesterone are slower to return in breast-feeding women. Lactation is initiated as levels of prolactin increase, and with increased breast-feeding the prolactin level rises further. In nonlactating women the prolactin level declines and reaches the pre-pregnancy level within 2 weeks postpartum. The extreme drop in hormones in the endocrine system allows two significant events to occur: lactation (milk secretion) begins with the newborn suckling, and the menstrual cycle function returns.

LACTATION

Postdelivery, estrogen, progesterone, and human placental lactogen (hPL) (all prolactin-inhibiting agents) decrease quickly, causing a quick increase in prolactin secretion.

- Once lactation has been established, suckling is the most important stimulus for the maintenance of milk production and ejection.
- Prolactin promotes milk production by stimulating the alveolar cells of the breast.
- Oxytocin, secreted by the posterior pituitary, triggers the ejection of milk as the newborn sucks. Oxytocin also stimulates uterine contractions (afterpains) felt by the mother.
- By the third postpartum day the prolactin effect on the breast tissue is apparent, and the hormone is present in sufficient quantity to cause breast engorgement.
- The breasts become distended, firm, tender, and warm. At this time, milk, which is thin and bluish, begins to replace the colostrum (premilk).
- If the mother does not wish to breast-feed her newborn, she should avoid any breast stimulation, including newborn suckling, pumping the breasts, or allowing warm water to flow on the breasts during showers.
- Prolactin levels drop quickly. Palpation of the breast on the second or third day will likely reveal engorgement—the breasts become distended (swollen), firm, tender, and warm to the touch due to vasocongestion.
- Breast **engorgement** is primarily caused by the temporary congestion of veins and lymphatics rather than by an accumulation of milk.
- Engorgement spontaneously resolves, and discomfort usually decreases within 24 to 36 hours. A snug, supportive bra worn for 72 hours; ice packs; and mild analgesics may be used to relieve breast discomfort.
- If suckling has never begun and nipple stimulation is avoided, lactation ceases within 3 to 7 days.

RESUMPTION OF OVULATION AND MENSTRUATION

- ❂ Most nonlactating mothers resume menstruation within 7 to 9 weeks after childbirth. Breast-feeding delays the return of ovulation and menstruation.
- ❂ Ovulation may return within 4 to 6 weeks in nonlactating women and up to 6 months in lactating women.
- ❂ Some lactating women do not menstruate as long as they nurse their newborns at least 10 to 12 times in a 24-hour period.
- ❂ The first menstrual flow is often greater than normal for both nursing and non-nursing mothers.
- ❂ The woman should be advised that it is possible to ovulate and become pregnant before her menstrual periods are established.

 Nurse Alert **Stress to the mother that breast-feeding is not an effective contraception method. The woman should be encouraged to discuss family planning with her health-care provider.**

WEIGHT LOSS

After delivery the mother's weight decreases by approximately 10 to 12 pounds. This weight loss is associated with the removal of the fetus, placenta, and amniotic fluid. An additional 5 pounds is lost during the early postpartum period as a result of diuresis and diaphoresis. During pregnancy the woman's body stores 5 to 7 pounds of adipose tissue for the energy requirements of labor and breast-feeding. The lactating mother gradually uses this fat store over the first 6 months, and she often returns to her approximate pre-pregnancy weight. Some women tend to retain some of the excess weight gained during pregnancy. Therefore, women are encouraged to perform postpartum exercises to lose the excess weight gained during pregnancy and increase the strength and tone of various muscles in their bodies. Aerobic exercise has no adverse effects on breast-feeding.

PSYCHOLOGICAL CHANGES

Mood swings (postpartum blues) are common during the postpartum period. The rapid decline of hormones such as progesterone and estrogen is believed to contribute to the emotional upset. Other factors related to emotional reactions are conflict about the maternal role and personal insecurity. Women who have economic or family problems usually demonstrate more stress in response to motherhood. In addition, past fetal losses or pregnancy failures contribute to postpartum emotional problems. Physical discomforts such as a painful perineum, afterpains, breast engorgement, and fatigue all contribute to negative postpartum reactions and should be promptly managed to promote comfort in the postpartum phase.

✔ ROUTINE CHECKUP 2

1. Why is the mother at risk for constipation? What interventions can be used to eliminate constipation?

Answer:

_____

_____

2. What are the complications associated with urinary retention?

Answer:

_____

_____

3. What interventions are used to increase the tone of the pubococcygeal muscle?

Answer:

_____

_____

4. What are the expected alterations in the cardiovascular system postdelivery?

Answer:

_____

_____

5. What factors increase the risk of postpartum blues?

Answer:

_____

_____

ROUTINE POSTPARTUM CARE

Providing safe, effective care to the new mother and infant can be challenging for many maternity nurses. Postpartum assessments begin during the fourth stage of labor and are complete with discharge (Table 11.3).

DISCHARGE CRITERIA

Most mothers leave the hospital as they are just beginning to recover from giving birth and learning how to care for themselves and the new infant. The nurse should confirm that the mother and significant others have understood discharge instructions. Discharge criteria include the following:

- ❍ The mother has no complications and the vital signs, lochia, fundus, urinary output, incisions, ambulation, ability to eat and drink, and emotional status are within normal parameters.

TABLE 11.3 • Postpartum Assessment and Care			
Assessment	First 8 Hours Postpartum	8 to 24 Hours Postpartum	24 to 48 Hours Postpartum
Vital signs	T., P., R., BP 1st hour: every 15 min 2nd hour: every 30 min 3rd to 8th hours: every 4 hours Monitor for hypotension and tachycardia. Note: After initial temperature evaluation, exclude T. from the every 15 min vital signs.	**Every 4 hours:** T., P., R., BP Monitor for hypotension and tachycardia. ↑ heart rate may be a sign of infection, pain, blood loss, or cardiac disease.	**Every 8 hours:** Continue assessment.
Skin color	Assess skin color, nail beds, and buccal cavity for abnormalities. 1st hour: every 15 min 2nd hour: every 30 min 3rd to 8th hours: every 4 hours	**Every 4 hours:** Assess skin color, nail beds, and buccal cavity for abnormalities.	**Every 8 hours:** Continue assessment.
Fundus assessment	Check location and tone. Ensure that the bladder is empty. If the fundus is soft or boggy, perform a fundal massage. Assess lochia with each massage. Do not massage the fundus if it is firm. 1st hour: every 15 min 2nd hour: every 30 min 3rd to 8th hours: every 4 hours	**Every 4 hours:** Check location and tone. Ensure that the bladder is empty. If the fundus is soft or boggy, perform a fundal massage. Assess lochia with each massage.	**Every 8 hours:** Continue assessment and nursing interventions.
Lochia	Assess for color, amount, odor, and clots on perineal pad. 1st hour: every 15 min 2nd hour: every 30 min 3rd to 8th hours: every 4 hours	**Every 4 hours:** Assess for color, amount, odor, and clots on perineal pad.	**Every 8 hours:** Continue assessment.

TABLE 11.3 • Postpartum Assessment and Care (*Continued*)			
Assessment	First 8 Hours Postpartum	8 to 24 Hours Postpartum	24 to 48 Hours Postpartum
Bladder assessment and urine output	Assess output amount, frequency, and discomfort. 1st hour: every 30 min 2nd hour: every hour 3rd to 8th hours: every 4 hours	**Every 4 hours:** Assess output amount, frequency, and discomfort.	**Every 8 hours:** Continue assessment.
Perineum	Assess for redness, edema, bruising, and discharge. If an episiotomy is present assess for approximation of the wound edges. 1st hour: every 30 min 2nd hour: every hour 3rd to 8th hours: every 8 hours Provide ice packs in the first 1–2 hours for swelling to the perineum. Then use heat lamp, sitz bath, astringents, topical analgesics, and pain medications as ordered. Administer stool softeners as needed. Encourage fluid intake and fiber intake to decrease constipation.	**Every 8 hours:** Assess for redness, edema, bruising, and discharge. If an episiotomy is present assess for approximation of the wound edges. Utilize appropriate nursing interventions to relieve discomfort. Administer stool softeners as needed. Encourage fluid intake and fiber intake to decrease constipation.	**Every 8 hours:** Continue assessment. Utilize appropriate nursing interventions to relieve discomfort. Administer stool softeners as needed.
Activity level	1st to 2nd hours: bed rest 3rd to 8th hours: Instruct patient to sit and dangle their feet over the side of the bed. Ensure stability. Up out of bed with assistance × 1, then up ad lib.	Up ad lib	Up ad lib. Instruct on abdominal breathing, head lifts, and modified sit-ups.

(Continued)

		8 to 24 Hours	24 to 48 Hours
Assessment	First 8 Hours Postpartum	Postpartum	Postpartum
Pain	**Pain assessment is the 5th vital sign.** 1st hour: every 15 min 2nd hour: every 30 min 3rd to 8th hours: every 4 hours Always assess pain at the appropriate interval after the administration of analgesics.	Every 4 hours and at the appropriate interval after administration of analgesics.	Every 4 hours and at the appropriate interval after administration of analgesics.
Breasts	**Assess every shift: size, symmetry, shape, softness, and nipple appearance.**	**Assess every shift.**	**Assess every shift.**
Rh factor	Check the prenatal and neonatal records to determine blood type and Rh factor to determine if RhoGAM should be administered. If the mother is Rh− and the newborn is RH+, and the mother is not already sensitized, Rh (D) immune globulin should be administered within 72 hours after delivery.		

TABLE 11.3 • Postpartum Assessment and Care (Continued)

◑ Hemoglobin and hematocrit have been reviewed, and immune globulin has been administered, if required.

◑ Instructions on self-care, normal postpartum symptoms, and abnormal postpartum symptoms have been reviewed with the mother verbalizing understanding.

◑ The mother demonstrates readiness to care for herself and the infant.

◑ Instructions on postpartum exercises, activity, and pain relief measures have been reviewed.

◑ Arrangement for postpartum care has been made.

◑ Support persons are available to the mother for at least 2 to 3 days post discharge.

Document teaching and evaluation of learning throughout the hospital stay and at discharge.

POSTPARTUM COMPLICATIONS

Pregnancy and childbirth are natural functions that most women recover from without complications. However, complications occur and nurses must be aware of the problems that may occur, their effect, and their treatment regimens.

POSTPARTUM HEMORRHAGE

What Went Wrong?

Postpartum hemorrhage is the most common cause of excessive bleeding during the childbearing cycle. Postpartum hemorrhage is traditionally defined as the loss of more than 500 mL of blood after an uncomplicated vaginal birth or 1000 mL after a cesarean birth. Because most women have 1 to 2 L of increased blood volume during pregnancy, they can tolerate this amount of blood loss. Postpartum hemorrhage can occur early (in the first 24 hours) or late (between 24 hours and 6 weeks after birth). The greatest danger, however, is in the first 24 hours because of the large venous area exposed after placental separation from the uterine wall. The most common causes of early postpartum hemorrhage are **uterine atony** and laceration. Late postpartum hemorrhage is caused by retained placental fragments or **subinvolution**.

Signs and Symptoms

- **Hypovolemia:** Increased heart and respiratory rates to increase the circulation of oxygenated red blood cells.
- Skin and mucous membranes are pale, cold, and moist.
- Blood flow to the brain decreases and the mother becomes restless, confused, anxious, and lethargic.

Nursing Management

A collaborative effort by the health-care team is necessary to provide prompt care. The management for hypovolemic shock (reduced blood volume) resulting from postpartum hemorrhage includes the following:

- Recognizing the specific cause (where the blood is coming from)
- Stopping the blood loss
- Starting intravenous fluids to maintain circulating volume
- Monitoring vital signs
- Providing oxygen to increase the saturation of red blood cells
- Inserting a Foley catheter to assess kidney function and urinary output

EARLY POSTPARTUM HEMORRHAGE

Risk Factors for Early Postpartum Hemorrhage

- Uterine atony
- Overdistention of the uterus
- Multifetal gestation
- Hydramnios

○ Oxytocin induction or augmentation
○ Lacerations
○ Bladder distention
○ Disseminated intravascular coagulation
○ Retained placental fragments

UTERINE ATONY

What Went Wrong?

Uterine atony (hypotonic uterus) is the most common cause of early post-partum hemorrhage. Uterine atony is the inability of the middle muscle, which has interlacing "figure eight" fibers of the uterus, to contract and stay contracted around the open blood vessels. Without this contraction, the vessels at the placental implantation site cannot close and begin to heal.

Mechanical factors that contribute to the inability of muscles to contract include retained placental fragments or large blood clots. Extreme uterine distention can cause uterine atony. Observation of a soft, boggy uterus that may be above the umbilicus is further evidence that bleeding is due to uterine atony. Overstretching may cause a lack of efficiency of the smooth muscle cells to contract. A full bladder can also prevent the uterus from contracting (Fig. 11.3).

Metabolic factors may contribute to uterine atony. Muscle exhaustion can occur from lactic acid buildup. Because calcium is an important regulator of smooth muscle tone, hypocalcemia may be implicated in some cases

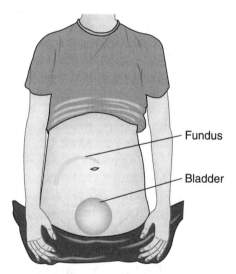

Figure 11.3 • Signs of hemorrhage: A distended bladder pushes the uterus upward and usually to one side of the abdomen. The fundus may be boggy or firm. If not emptied, a distended bladder can result in uterine atony and hemorrhage because it interferes with the normal contraction of the uterus.

of uterine atony. Drugs have important effects on postpartum uterine tone. Magnesium sulfate administered to prevent seizures or as a tocolytic agent may result in uterine atony by impairing calcium-mediated properties within the cells. In addition, calcium channel blockers, such as nifedipine, used in preterm uterine contractions may also inhibit postpartum uterine contractions.

Signs and Symptoms

- Fundus that is difficult to locate
- A soft or "boggy feeling" fundus
- A uterus that becomes firm with massage but loses its tone when the massage is stopped
- Excessive lochia that is bright red
- Excessive clots are expelled

Treatments

- Bimanual compression of the uterus if nursing interventions and oxytocin are ineffective
- Possible return to the operating room for exploration of the uterus cavity and removal of placental fragments

Nursing Interventions

To decrease the risk of uterine atony, the nurse should do the following:

- Ensure the bladder is empty.
- Assess the fundus for firmness and position.
- Massage the uterus if necessary to increase tone.
- Assess and monitor lochia flow; report abnormal bleeding or excessive clots.
- Monitor the mother's vital signs and inability of the uterus to contract.
- If uterine atony is suspected the nurse should prepare for baseline laboratory studies (complete blood count [CBC] and coagulation profile) and intravenous therapy with dextran or albumin and blood products. High doses of oxytocin (Pitocin) may be indicated.

HEMATOMA

What Went Wrong?

Hematoma is the collection of blood within the tissues, which may result from injury to blood vessels in the perineum or in the vagina. Soft tissues in other areas may be involved, which are typically seen as a bulging, bluish mass. Hematomas containing 250 to 500 mL of blood may develop rapidly. A hematoma may form in the upper segment of the vagina or may occur upward into the broad ligament, which can result in substantial hemorrhage.

Perineal pain, rather than noticeable bleeding, is a distinctive feature of a hematoma, and the uterus remains firm. The mother may not be able to void because of pressure on the urethra, or she may feel the urge to defecate because of pressure on the rectum.

Treatments

- Return the mother to labor and delivery for surgical incision to remove the clot.
- Small vulvar hematomas may be treated with application of ice packs or alternate hot and cold applications.

Nursing Interventions

- Don gloves and inspect the perineum.
- Report any visualized hematoma.
- Monitor lochia flow, amount, and color.
- Assess pain: Hematomas produce intense, deep pain and a feeling of pressure.
- Monitor vital signs for increased pulse rate and decreased BP.
- Prepare the mother for surgery if needed.

LATE POSTPARTUM HEMORRHAGE

What Went Wrong?

Late postpartum hemorrhage can occur 1 to 2 weeks after delivery and is typically due to **subinvolution**, which is defined as failure of the uterus to return to pre-pregnancy size. The site of placental implantation is the last to heal and regenerate after delivery. A vascular area, retained placental fragments, or infection may be the cause of late postpartum hemorrhage.

Signs and Symptoms

- A fundal height higher than expected postpartum.
- Persistent lochia rubra.
- Irregular or excessive bleeding.
- Uterus that is larger than normal and may be boggy.
- Infection may be suspected if a foul odor to the lochia is noted.

Treatments

- Treatment is tailored to correct the cause of the subinvolution.
- Antibiotics may be needed if an infection is present.
- The mother may require methylergonovine maleate.

Nursing Interventions

- Patient teaching on locating and palpating the fundus and estimating fundus height is extremely important since subinvolution of the uterus generally occurs after the mother is home.
- Explain that the uterus should become smaller each day.
- Explain differences in lochia flow: amount, color, consistency, and smell.
- Instruct the mother to report fundal pain, foul smelling vaginal drainage, and any deviation from the expected lochia flow.

☑ ROUTINE CHECKUP 3

1. What are the signs and symptoms of uterine atony?
Answer:

2. What nursing interventions decrease the risk of uterine atony?
Answer:

3. What are the major signs of uterine subinvolution?
Answer:

4. What are the nursing interventions to manage subinvolution?
Answer:

DISSEMINATED INTRAVASCULAR COAGULATION

What Went Wrong?

Disseminated intravascular coagulation (DIC) is a condition in which clotting and anticoagulation stimulation occur at the same time. The release of thromboplastin uses up available fibrinogen and platelets, which results in profuse bleeding and intravascular clotting. The key to the successful management of DIC is treatment of the causative event. It often is a secondary condition associated with abruptio placenta, gestational hypertension, missed abortion, or fetal death in utero. DIC is suspected when the usual measures to stimulate uterine contractions fail to stop vaginal bleeding.

Signs and Symptoms

- Oozing from an intravenous insertion site
- Petechiae
- Ecchymosis
- Oliguria
- Restlessness
- Decreasing pulse pressure with continued bleeding

ASSESSMENT AND MANAGEMENT OF POSTPARTUM HEMORRHAGE

Signs and Symptoms

- Boggy uterus
- Uterine fundus above the umbilicus
- Excessive lochia
- Fundus displaced
- Tachycardia
- Hypotension
- Change in level of consciousness

Test Results

- Hemoglobin and hematocrit: Level is reduced.
- Fibrin: Level is reduced.
- Platelet count: Level is reduced.
- Type and cross-match.
- D-dimer: Increased.
- Arterial blood gases: Oxygen saturation is decreased.
- Coagulation profile: Prolonged and increased.
  - Prothrombin time (PT)
  - Partial thromboplastin time (PTT)

Treatments

- Intravenous therapy with dextran or albumin and blood products.
- High doses of oxytocin (Pitocin) may be indicated.
- Treatment may include administration of methylergonovine (Methergine) orally or intramuscularly to contract the uterus.
- Recombinant-activated factor VIIa given intravenously for reversal of symptoms of DIC.
- Antimicrobials if infection is present.
- The physician may use bimanual compression by placing one hand in the vagina with the other pushing against the fundus through the abdominal wall to control bleeding.
- Dilatation and evacuation if retained placental fragments are suspected.

 Nurse Alert **Treatment consists of the administration of methylergonovine. Methylergonovine may be contraindicated in hypertensive women.**

Nursing Interventions

Prevention of Hemorrhage

Postpartum hemorrhage caused by uterine atony after a vaginal birth can be greatly reduced by the following:

- Prophylactic administration of uterotonic drugs (oxytocin) after the delivery of the placenta. An intravenous solution of oxytocin may be started to contract the uterus.

- ◐ Early clamping of the umbilical cord and assisted delivery of the placenta may also prevent uterine atony and postpartum hemorrhage.
- ◐ The nurse should prepare for baseline laboratory studies.
- ◐ Administration of vitamin K assists with endogenous replenishment of factors II, VII, IX, and X, which aid in blood clotting. Recombinant-activated factor VIIa in an intravenous solution can reverse the symptoms of disseminated intravascular coagulation.

Management of Postpartum Hemorrhage

- ◐ Uterine massage (avoid potential uterine inversion): Avoid excessively vigorous massage of the uterus, which could increase the risk of subinvolution.
- ◐ Maintenance of large-bore intravenous catheters.
- ◐ Administration of intravenous fluids (e.g., rapid volume expanders, blood products).
- ◐ Foley catheter (to maintain accurate measurement of urine output): Urinary output should be at least 30 mL/h.
- ◐ Pulse oximeter use and saturation level monitoring.
- ◐ Administration of oxygen (per protocol).
- ◐ Elevation of legs at a 20- to 30-degree angle to increase venous return.
- ◐ Avoid the use of the Trendelenburg position (unless ordered), since it may interfere with cardiac and respiratory function.
- ◐ Explain procedures to the mother (why they are necessary).
- ◐ Provide emotional support for the mother and her family.
- ◐ Assess blood loss by weighing the perineal pads (1g of pad weight = 1ml (cc) blood loss volume, subtracting the weight of dry pad from saturated pad). If possible, a gram scale should be kept in the postpartum unit and used to measure blood loss.
- ◐ Monitor vital signs every 15 minutes until stabilized.

THROMBOPHLEBITIS AND THROMBOEMBOLISM

Thrombophlebitis is inflammation of the inner blood vessel wall with a blood clot attached to that wall. A **thrombus** is a blood clot obstructing a blood vessel that remains at the place that it was formed. When the blood clot tears away and moves into the circulation, it is called an *embolus*. If the embolus lands in the lung, it is called a pulmonary embolus—a common postpartum complication. Thrombophlebitis can be superficial and involve saphenous or surface veins, or it may be deep (deep vein thrombosis [DVT]) and involve the deep venous system from the foot to the iliofemoral region.

What Went Wrong?

All postpartum women are at high risk for thrombophlebitis because of the normal hypercoagulability of the blood at delivery that prevents hemorrhage, venous stasis from pressure of the gravid uterus, and inactivity. Approximately 50% of thromboembolism is associated with inherited thrombophilia. Screening or prophylactic measures for those at inherited risk have not yet been established.

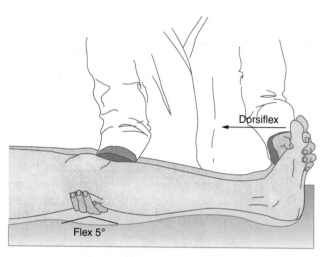

Figure 11.4 • Homans' sign is positive when the mother has discomfort on sharp dorsiflexion of the foot. A positive Homans' sign should be promptly reported. (Gabbe, Niebyl, & Simpson, 2007)

Assessment

The nurse, in a routine postpartum assessment, may be the first person to identify signs of thromboembolic disorders. The nurse may note subjective signs of pain when she palpates the calves of the legs for heat and tenderness. Pain in the calf when the foot is passively dorsiflexed is called a positive **Homans' sign** (Fig. 11.4). However, DVT can be present despite a negative Homans' sign. Comparison of pulses in both extremities may reveal decreased blood flow to the affected area. Serial measurements of the affected extremity will reveal an increased diameter (edema and swelling) caused by venous inflammation. Leg pain that extends above the knee may indicate DVT. Fever and chills may occur.

Risk Factors for Thrombophlebitis
- Ceasarean birth
- Varicose veins
- Decreased activity
- Diabetes mellitus
- Smoking
- Obesity
- History of thrombophlebitis
- Prolonged standing or sitting
- Parity >3
- Maternal age >35
- Inactivity

Signs and Symptoms

- Swelling of extremity
- Decreased pulses to affected extremity
- Positive Homans' sign
- Erythema and pain to affected site
- Pedal edema

Diagnostic Evaluation

- Computed tomography
- Magnetic resonance angiography
- Ultrasound
- Duplex scanning

Laboratory Tests

- Coagulation studies

Nursing Interventions

- Management for superficial venous thrombosis includes bed rest.
- Gradual ambulation with decreased symptoms and anticoagulant therapy.
- Antiembolism stockings.
- Analgesics for comfort.
- Elevation of the leg.
- Anticoagulation therapy is started with intravenous heparin administered by continuous intravenous infusion.
- Heat to the affected extremity.

 Nurse Alert **Doses of heparin are adjusted according to partial thromboplastin time (PTT). While the mother is receiving heparin therapy, her platelet count must be monitored closely. The activated partial thromboplastin time (aPTT) should be monitored, and the heparin dose should be adjusted to maintain a therapeutic level of 1.5 to 2.5 times control.**

- Measures to prevent thrombophlebitis should be part of every teaching plan throughout pregnancy and postpartum. Early ambulation, avoidance of prolonged sitting and crossing of legs, elevation of legs when possible, and adequate hydration are important preventive measures.
- Measures to prevent thrombophlebitis:
    - Avoid prolonged standing or sitting.
    - Elevate legs when sitting.
    - Avoid crossing legs (will reduce circulation and encourage venous stasis).
    - Exercise to improve circulation (e.g., walking).
    - Maintain 2500 mL (2.5 quarts) of fluid intake per day.
    - Prevent dehydration, which encourages sluggish circulation.
    - Stop smoking (a known risk factor).

✓ ROUTINE CHECKUP 4

1. What factors place the new mother at greater risk for thrombophlebitis?
Answer:

_____

_____

2. What are the signs and symptoms of thrombophlebitis?
Answer:

_____

_____

PULMONARY EMBOLISM

WHAT WENT WRONG?

Pulmonary embolism is reported as one of the three leading causes of maternal death, along with hemorrhage and gestational hypertension, and is a feared complication of DVT. It occurs when fragments of a blood clot dislodge and are carried to the pulmonary artery or one of its branches. The embolism can occlude the vessel and obstruct the flow of blood into the lungs. If the pulmonary circulation is severely compromised, death may occur in minutes.

SIGNS AND SYMPTOMS

- Chills
- Hypotension
- Dyspnea
- Sharp chest pain
- Tachypnea
- Apprehension
- Syncope
- Hemoptysis

DIAGNOSTIC EVALUATION

- Pulse oximetry
- Chest radiography
- Ventilation-perfusion scan

TREATMENTS

- Treatment measures to dissolve the clot (anticoagulants).
- An embolectomy (surgical removal of the embolus) may be required.

NURSING INTERVENTIONS

○ Immediate medical and nursing interventions include raising the head of the bed to facilitate breathing.

○ Administer oxygen by mask.

○ Anticoagulation therapy is started with intravenous heparin administered by continuous intravenous infusion.

○ Prepare the mother for transfer to the critical care unit for critical care nursing.

POSTPARTUM (PUERPERAL) INFECTION

Postpartum infection still accounts for significant rates of postpartum maternal morbidity and mortality. Postpartum infections fall into two broad categories. The first covers reproductive system infections (**puerperal infection**), which are bacterial infections that arise in the genital tract after delivery. The second category includes non–reproductive system infections that arise in sites other than the genital tract and influence maternal morbidity during the postpartum recovery phase. These infections, which include mastitis and urinary tract infections, are indirectly related to the physiologic features of pregnancy, labor, birth, and lactation. A woman is considered to have a puerperal infection if she has a fever of 38°C (100.4°F) or higher after the first 24 hours following delivery and the fever is maintained for at least 2 days within the first 10 days postpartum.

WHAT WENT WRONG?

The uterus and cervix are open after delivery of the fetus and are exposed through the vagina to the external environment. Exposed blood vessels are well supplied, and wounds from lacerations or incisions may be present; therefore, the risk of microorganisms entering the reproductive tract and extending into the blood and other parts of the body is high, which could result in life-threatening septicemia.

Normal physiologic changes that occur during pregnancy increase the risk of infection. During labor, amniotic fluid, blood, and lochia, which are alkaline, decrease the acidity of the vagina; therefore, the vaginal environment encourages the growth of pathogens. Many small lacerations occur in the endometrium, cervix, and vagina, which allow pathogens to enter the tissues.

A cesarean birth is a major predisposing factor and poses a greater risk than a vaginal birth for postpartum infection. This is because of the trauma to tissues during surgery and the fact that many of these women have other risks, such as prolonged labor. When premature rupture of membranes occurs, organisms from the vagina are more likely to ascend into the uterine cavity and increase the risk of infection. Each vaginal examination increases the risk of pathogens entering the vagina and, in effect, being pushed into the cervix. As the area of placental attachment heals, necrotic tissue develops, which provides an ideal medium for bacterial growth.

SIGNS AND SYMPTOMS

- Fever, tachycardia, chills (temperature greater than 38°C [100.4°F]).
- Uterine tenderness.
- Localized reddened, warm, and tender area.
- Purulent wound drainage.
- Lochia: Appearance varies depending on causative organism; may be normal, profuse, scant, foul smelling.
- Uterine subinvolution (uterus boggy, soft fundus, location higher than normal).
- Malaise.

LABORATORY TESTS

- CBC
- Blood cultures
- Urine culture
- Vaginal cultures

NURSING INTERVENTIONS

- Assess temperature at least every 4 hours, and within 45 minutes to 1 hour after administering antipyretics.
- Administer antipyretics.
- Administer antibiotics.
- Teach proper peritoneal care.
- Monitor lochia.

 ROUTINE CHECKUP 5

1. What factors increase the risk for postpartum infection in mothers who had a cesarean birth?

Answer:

_____
_____

2. Identify the normal physiologic changes of childbearing that make a mother susceptible to infection of the reproductive system.

Answer:

_____
_____

ENDOMETRITIS

Endometritis (also called metritis) is the most common postpartum infection. It is an infection of the endometrial lining and adjacent myometrium of the uterus. Symptoms begin on the second to fifth day postpartum. This condition affects approximately 3% of women delivering vaginally and 10% to 30% of those delivering by cesarean birth. Endometritis, if untreated, can quickly progress to **parametritis** (infection spread by lymphatics through the uterine wall to the broad ligament or the entire pelvis) and can spread, causing peritonitis and possibly a pelvic abscess.

SIGNS AND SYMPTOMS

- Onset usually 24 hours after delivery
- Uterine tenderness and enlargement
- Foul odor or purulent lochia that may increase or decrease in amount
- Malaise, fatigue, tachycardia
- Temperature elevation

LABORATORY TESTS

- CBC
- Blood cultures
- Urine culture
- Vaginal cultures

NURSING INTERVENTIONS

- Assess temperature at least every 4 hours and within 45 minutes to 1 hour after administering antipyretics.
- Administer antipyretics.
- Administer antibiotics.
- Teach proper peritoneal care.
- Monitor lochia amount and color.
- Place mother in Fowler's position to promote drainage of lochia.
- Administer analgesics as needed for pain.

WOUND INFECTION

Wound infections are common types of puerperal infections because of the many sites involving any break in the skin or mucous membrane. The most common sites are the perineum, where episiotomies and lacerations are located, and the cesarean surgical incision. Multiple vaginal examinations also increase the risk of infection.

NURSING ASSESSMENT

- Assess the perineal area for redness, swelling, bruising, and wound approximation.
- Assess for drainage and odor.
- Note lochia color and amount.
- Assess for signs of infection such as fever and malaise.

SIGNS AND SYMPTOMS

- Redness at the incision site
- Edema at the incision site
- Ecchymosis at the incision site
- Discharge at the incision site
- Pain
- Fever and malaise

LABORATORY TESTS

- Blood cultures
- Urine cultures
- CBC

TREATMENT

- Incision and drainage of affected area may be necessary.

NURSING INTERVENTIONS

- If the mother requires surgery monitor the surgical site and perform perineal care. The wound may be packed with sterile gauze if débridement is necessary. Removing packing and repacking the wound become part of the care provided to the mother.
- Administer analgesics as ordered.
- Warm compresses and sitz baths may soothe the painful perineal area.
- Teach proper perineal care and hand washing technique.

MASTITIS

Mastitis (infection of the breasts) usually occurs approximately 2 to 3 weeks after birth and may occur as early as the seventh postpartum day. The infection involves the interlobular connective tissue, usually involving one breast.

WHAT WENT WRONG?

Predisposing factors include milk stasis (from a blocked duct), nipple trauma (cracked or fissured nipples), and poor breast-feeding technique. Other causes of mastitis are inadequate hand washing between handling perineal pads and then the breasts.

SIGNS AND SYMPTOMS

- Painful or tender, localized, hard mass and reddened area, usually of one breast.
- The woman may also have enlarged glands in the axilla on the affected side.
- Fever, chills, and malaise may accompany the infection and, if untreated, it may progress into an abscess.

NURSING INTERVENTIONS

- Antibiotics.
- To prevent stasis of milk, the breasts must be completely emptied at each feeding. This can be done every 11/2 to 2 hours to make the mother more comfortable and prevent stasis.
- The woman is encouraged to wear a well-supporting, properly fitted brassiere.
- To relieve discomfort, she can use ice or warm packs (whichever feels better). Moist heat promotes comfort and increases circulation.
- To prevent mastitis, the woman should be taught breast hygiene, how to prevent breast engorgement, adequate breast support, proper hand hygiene, and breast-feeding techniques.

SELF-CARE FOR MASTITIS

- Wash hands thoroughly before breast-feeding.
- Maintain breast cleanliness with frequent breast pad change.
- Expose nipples to air.
- Correct newborn latch-on and removal from breast.
- Encourage the newborn to empty the breast because milk provides a medium for bacterial growth.
- Frequently breast-feed to encourage milk flow.
- If an area of the breast is distended or tender, breast-feed from the uninfected side first at each feeding (to initiate the let-down reflex in the affected breast).
- Massage the distended area as the newborn nurses.
- Report redness and fever.
- Apply ice packs or moist heat to relieve discomfort.

URINARY TRACT INFECTION

◢◣ WHAT WENT WRONG?

Urinary tract infection can occur after birth from hypotonia of the bladder, urinary stasis, birth trauma, catheterization, frequent vaginal examinations, or epidural anesthesia. During birth the bladder and urethra can be traumatized by pressure from the descending fetus. After birth a hypotonic bladder and urethra can increase both urinary stasis and urinary retention.

SIGNS AND SYMPTOMS

- Cystitis (inflammation of urinary bladder)
- Pyelonephritis (inflammation of kidney)
- Urinary urgency
- Urinary frequency
- Suprapubic pain
- Dysuria
- Hematuria (not always present)
- Fever, chills
- Costovertebral angle tenderness
- Leukocytosis
- Nausea and vomiting

NURSING INTERVENTIONS

- Monitor vital signs every 4 hours.
- Encourage increased fluid intake to dilute the bacterial count and flush the infection from the bladder.
- Encourage intake of cranberry juice to increase the acidification of the urine, which inhibits multiplication of bacteria.
- Teach perineal hygiene and ensure that the woman recognizes the need to wipe the perineum from the front to the back, and to wear cotton underclothing.
- Antispasmodic or urinary analgesic agents, such as phenazopyridine hydrochloride (Pyridium), may be prescribed to relieve bladder discomfort.

POSTPARTUM DEPRESSION

WHAT WENT WRONG?

Postpartum blues, postpartum depression, and postpartum psychosis are not part of a continuum of the same disorder. The symptoms may be similar, but the conditions are different.

The signs of **postpartum depression (PPD)** include general signs of depression such as weight loss, sleeplessness, and ambivalence toward the newborn and family. Postpartum depression occurs in approximately 13% of new mothers and may have long-term effects on mother-newborn interaction.

Symptoms of postpartum depression may be evident before hospital discharge, and patients at risk should be scheduled for follow-up visits before the traditional 6-week postpartum visit. Women at high risk for postpartum depression have risk factors such as:

- ◑ Unstable or abusive family environment
- ◑ History of previous depressive episode
- ◑ History of limited support system
- ◑ Low self-esteem
- ◑ Dissatisfaction with education, economics, or choice of partner

POSTPARTUM PSYCHOSIS

The symptoms of postpartum psychosis are similar to those of other psychoses.

SIGNS AND SYMPTOMS

Early signs of depression may be evident, or they may start abruptly within 3 weeks after childbirth:

- ◑ Confusion.
- ◑ Restlessness.
- ◑ Anxiety.
- ◑ Suicidal thoughts may occur.
- ◑ Delusional thoughts may be expressed.
- ◑ The woman and her newborn are at risk for their safety.

TREATMENT

Psychiatric supervision is necessary, and antipsychotic medications with the addition of sublingual estradiol may be prescribed (Gabbe, Niebyl, & Simpson, 2007).

NURSING INTERVENTIONS

- ◑ Encourage expression of feelings.
- ◑ Validate the mother's emotions.

CONCLUSION

Pregnancy and childbirth are natural functions that most women recuperate from without complications. The postpartum period is the 6-week interval from childbirth to the return of the uterus and other organs to a pre-pregnancy state. The main goals in postpartum care are to assist and support the mother's recovery to the pre-pregnancy state and identify deviations from the norm. To provide high-quality care, the nurse must be knowledgeable about the physical and emotional physiology of postpartum adaptation. After the initial dangers of **hemorrhage** and **shock** have passed, the primary postpartum danger is **infection**. The uterine cavity is easily accessible to microorganisms from the exterior. Also, the site where the placenta was attached is an open wound and can be easily infected.

- Postpartum hemorrhage is blood loss exceeding 500 mL in a vaginal delivery and 1000 mL in a cesarean birth. Hemorrhage may occur early or late in the postpartum period.
- Leading causes of early postpartum hemorrhage are uterine atony, lacerations, and retained placental fragments.
- The leading cause of delayed hemorrhage is subinvolution of the uterus, which may result from retained tissue fragments.
- Thromboembolic disorders can complicate the postpartum period. Changes in the blood coagulation system during the postpartum period place the woman at risk for thromboembolic conditions such as superficial venous thrombophlebitis and DVT.
- A life-threatening complication is pulmonary embolism, which requires immediate intensive care. Pulmonary embolism, although not common, is reported as a major cause of maternal death. It occurs when fragments of a blood clot dislodge, are carried to a pulmonary artery, and block the flow of blood into the lungs.
- Puerperal infections involving the reproductive system account for many complications in the postpartum period. Two common postpartum infections are mastitis and urinary tract infection.

? FINAL CHECKUP

1. **A woman who has recently given birth complains of pain and tenderness in her leg. Upon physical examination, the nurse notices warmth and redness over an enlarged, hardened area. The nurse should suspect _____ and should confirm the diagnosis by _____.**
   a. disseminated intravascular coagulation ... asking for laboratory tests
   b. von Willebrand disease ... noting whether bleeding times have been extended
   c. thrombophlebitis ... using real-time and color Doppler ultrasound
   d. coagulopathies ... drawing blood for laboratory analysis

2. **A woman gave birth to an infant boy 10 hours ago. Where would the nurse expect to locate this woman's fundus?**
   a. One centimeter above the umbilicus
   b. Two centimeters below the umbilicus
   c. Midway between the umbilicus and the symphysis pubis
   d. Nonpalpable abdominally

3. **The most common causes of subinvolution are which of the following?**
   a. Postpartum hemorrhage and infection
   b. Multiple gestation and postpartum hemorrhage
   c. Uterine tetany and overproduction of oxytocin
   d. Retained placental fragments and infection

4. A woman gave birth to a healthy infant boy 5 days ago. What type of lochia would the nurse expect to find when assessing this woman?
   a. Lochia rubra
   b. Lochia sangra
   c. Lochia alba
   d. Lochia serosa

5. Nurses should be aware of which of the following with regard to the postpartum uterus?
   a. At the end of the third stage of labor, it weighs approximately 500 g.
   b. After 2 weeks postpartum, it should not be palpable abdominally.
   c. After 2 weeks postpartum, it weighs 100 g.
   d. It returns to its original (pre-pregnancy) size by 6 weeks postpartum.

6. On examining a woman who gave birth 5 hours ago, the nurse finds that the woman has completely saturated a perineal pad within 15 minutes. The nurse's first action is to do what?
   a. Begin an intravenous (IV) infusion of Ringer's lactate solution.
   b. Assess the woman's vital signs.
   c. Call the woman's primary health-care provider.
   d. Massage the woman's fundus.

7. If a woman is at risk for thrombus and is not ready to ambulate, nurses might intervene by doing all of the following *except* what?
   a. Putting her in TED hose and/or SCD boots
   b. Having her flex, extend, and rotate her feet, ankles, and legs
   c. Having her sit in a chair
   d. Notifying the physician immediately if a positive Homans' sign occurs

8. A primary nursing responsibility when caring for a woman experiencing an obstetric hemorrhage associated with uterine atony is to do what?
   a. Establish venous access.
   b. Perform fundal massage.
   c. Prepare the woman for surgical intervention.
   d. Catheterize the bladder.

9. The most effective and least expensive treatment of puerperal infection is prevention. Which of the following is important in this strategy?
   a. Large doses of vitamin C during pregnancy
   b. Prophylactic antibiotics
   c. Strict aseptic technique, including hand washing, by all health care personnel
   d. Limited protein and fat intake

10. **In caring for an immediately postpartum client, you note petechiae and oozing from her IV site. You would monitor her closely for which clotting disorder?**
   a. Disseminated intravascular coagulation
   b. Amniotic fluid embolism
   c. Hemorrhage
   d. HELLP syndrome

References

Blackburn ST. (2003). *Maternal, Fetal, and Neonatal Physiology*. 2nd ed. Philadelphia: Saunders.

Gabbe SG, Niebyl JR, & Simpson, JL. (2007). *Obstetrics: Normal and Problem Pregnancies*. 5th ed. Philadelphia: Elsevier Churchill Livingstone.

Lowdermilk DL, Perry SE, Alden KR, Cashion K, & Corbett RW. (2006). *Maternity Nursing*. 7th ed. St. Louis, MO: Mosby Elsevier.

ANSWERS

Routine Checkup 1

1. During the fourth stage of labor the nursing priority is given to the assessment of the mother for signs and symptoms of postpartum hemorrhage. The mother's skin color, level of consciousness, fundus firmness, lochia flow, bladder, activity level, and vital signs (excluding temperature) should be assessed every 15 minutes.
2. Involution.
3. Lochia rubra is characterized as red vaginal flow consisting mostly of blood, but also having small clots and a fleshy odor, and occurs during the first 1 to 3 days postpartum. Lochia serosa is characterized as serous, pink or brownish, watery vaginal flow occurring during the 4th through the 10th day postpartum. Lochia alba is identified as creamy white or light yellow vaginal discharge, which occurs around postpartum day 11 and may last for 6 weeks.
4. The nurse should use the following interventions to relieve perineal discomfort post-delivery: Use aseptic technique and don gloves for perineal care; teach appropriate technique for perineal care (wipe from front to back); teach the mother how to perform a sitz bath; instruct the mother on the use of topical anesthetics and astringent pads if ordered; and assess pain level and administer analgesics as needed.

Routine Checkup 2

1. Constipation is commonly a problem during the postpartum period because of the following:
   (a) Decreased peristalsis caused by the remaining relaxing effects of progesterone
   (b) Stretched abdominal muscles, which make it difficult to bear down to expel stool
   (c) Soreness and swelling of the perineum and hemorrhoids
   (d) Fear of pain

Interventions to eliminate constipation include administering stool softeners or laxatives, increasing fluid intake, and increasing activity.

2. Urinary retention and over-distention of the bladder may lead to urinary tract infection and postpartum hemorrhage.

3. Encourage Kegel exercises to help the pubococcygeal muscle to regain normal function.

4. An initial increase in cardiac output post birth caused by an increase in blood flow back to the heart from the elimination of the placenta, which diverts 500 to 750 mL of blood flow into the maternal systemic circulation, and a rapid decrease in the size of the uterus, which decreases pressure on the vessels.

   Also, changes are related to the movement of excess extracellular fluid into the vascular compartment.

5. The rapid decline of hormones such as progesterone and estrogen is believed to contribute to the emotional upset. Other factors related to emotional reactions are conflict about the maternal role and personal insecurity. Women who have economic or family problems usually demonstrate more stress in response to motherhood. In addition, past fetal losses or pregnancy failures contribute to postpartum emotional problems. Physical discomforts such as a painful perineum, afterpains, breast engorgement, and fatigue all contribute to negative postpartum reactions.

Routine Checkup 3

1. Signs and symptoms of uterine atony are boggy or displaced uterus that may be above the umbilicus; tachycardia is further evidence that bleeding is due to uterine atony.

2. To decrease the risk of uterine atony, the nurse should assess the fundus and massage if necessary to increase tone and ensure that the bladder is empty. Monitor the mother's vital signs and report abnormal bleeding and the inability of the uterus to contract. If uterine atony is suspected the nurse should prepare for baseline laboratory studies and intravenous therapy with dextran or albumin and blood products. High doses of oxytocin (Pitocin) may be ordered by the physician.

3. Signs and symptoms include prolonged lochial discharge, irregular or excessive bleeding, and sometimes hemorrhage. A pelvic examination usually reveals a uterus that is larger than normal and that may be boggy.

4. Patient teaching on locating and palpating the fundus and estimating its height is extremely important since subinvolution of the uterus generally occurs after the mother is home. Explain differences in lochia flow: amount, color, consistency, and smell. The nurse should explain that the uterus should become smaller each day. Instruct the mother to report fundal pain, foul smelling vaginal drainage, and any deviation from the expected lochia flow.

Routine Checkup 4

1. All postpartum women are at high risk for thrombophlebitis because of the normal hypercoagulability of the blood at delivery that prevents hemorrhage, venous stasis from pressure of the gravid uterus, and inactivity.
2. Swelling of extremity, decreased pulses to affected extremity, positive Homans' sign, erythema to the affected site, pedal edema, and pain at the affected site.

Routine Checkup 5

1. A cesarean birth is a major predisposing factor and poses a greater risk than a vaginal birth for postpartum infection. This is because of the trauma to tissues during surgery and the fact that many of these women have other risks, such as prolonged labor.
2. During labor, amniotic fluid, blood, and lochia, which are alkaline, decrease the acidity of the vagina; therefore, the vaginal environment encourages the growth of pathogens. Many small lacerations occur in the endometrium, cervix, and vagina, which allow pathogens to enter the tissues. As the area of placental attachment heals, necrotic tissue develops, which provides an ideal medium for bacterial growth.

Final Checkup

1. c	2. a	3. d	4. d	5. b
6. d	7. c	8. b	9. c	10. a

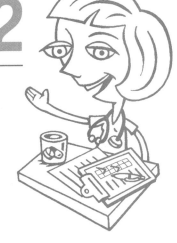

CHAPTER **12**

Newborn Care

Objectives

At the end of this chapter, the student will be able to:

1. Review the changes that occur during the newborn period and related care.

2. Evaluate assessments and diagnostic findings associated with the newborn.

3. Discuss health promotion interventions that promote family and newborn adjustment.

4. Teach and support parents and families regarding the care required for a newborn.

5. Discuss congenital and other conditions that threaten newborn health and well-being.

 KEY TERMS

Caput succedaneum	Hypoglycemia
Cephalhematoma	Pathologic jaundice
Extrauterine life	Phototherapy
Galactosemia	Physiologic jaundice
Hyperbilirubinemia	Respiratory distress syndrome
Hyperglycemia	

IMMEDIATE CARE AFTER BIRTH

The newborn requires an immediate and thorough skilled assessment to ensure a satisfactory adjustment to extrauterine life. As stated in Chapter 10, the nose and mouth are suctioned when the head is born. The umbilical cord is clamped and cut, and then the baby is placed on the mother's chest for initial contact. The nurse should observe and note if the cord has two arteries and one vein (altered cord circulation could indicate oxygen or nutrient deficit in utero). A focused assessment of Apgar scoring, temperature stability, level of reactivity, size for gestational age, and attachment behaviors should be performed. A system's approach assessment occurs immediately after birth.

Temperature stability: Support measures are provided to maintain body heat. The newborn is dried and wrapped in blankets or warmed against the mother's skin to allow early bonding and breast-feeding, if desired. If a radiant warmer is used, the newborn is left uncovered for direct heating of the skin.

Apgar scoring is done at 1 minute after birth and repeated at 5 mintes after birth. A score of 0 to 2 is assigned to each area assessed (see Table 12.1).

Level of reactivity is determined by newborn response, or lack of response, to stimuli. Generally newborns will have an initial period of reactivity immediately after birth. During this period the newborn will be alert with increased respiratory rate and heart rate, strong sucking motions, and bouts of random movement alternating with stillness. After about 30 minutes of reactivity the newborn enters a sleep phase that lasts from 2 to 4 hours. After the sleep period the newborn has a second period of reactivity that may last from 4 to 6 hours. The periods of reactivity are ideal times to initiate breast-feeding if desired, and to promote bonding between the newborn and family.

Gestational age is assessed based on physical characteristics and neuro-muscular development. Initial assessment may be done in the first hour and a repeat assessment is done 24 hours later to capture those reflexes and other neurologic findings that were unstable for the first 24 hours. New Ballard

TABLE 12.1 • Apgar test score criteria			
Criterion	0	1	2
Heart rate	Absent	slow, <100 beats per minute	>100
Respiratory effort	Absent	Slow, irregular	Good cry
Muscle tone	Flaccid	Flexion of extremities	Active movement noted
Reflex irritability	None	Grimace noted	Strong cry
Color	Pallor or blue skin undertones	Pink/red body; blue extremities (acrocyanosis)	All skin pink/red undertones

Score (NBS) or Dubowitz tools may be used to assess gestational age. The primary areas of assessment include the following:

Neuromuscular maturity:

- Posture (term newborn lies with flexion of extremities)
- Wrist (square window >90-degree flexion in preterm → 0 flexion if term)
- Arm recoil (<90-degree flexion angle if term)
- Popliteal angle (180 degrees for preterm to <90 degrees for term)
- Scarf sign (preterm's elbow pulls past the midline of the body without resistance)
- Heel to ear (premature infant can pull heels to ear)

Physical maturity:

- Skin (sticky, transparent, fragile in preterm → leathery, cracked in post-term)
- Lanugo (none in extreme preterm, heavy in mid-preterm, none in post-term)
- Plantar surface (creases over full sole of foot in term infant)
- Breast (not notable in preterm—clear areola with 5–10 mm bud)
- Eye/ear (preterm eyelids fused loosely/tightly → eyes open; thick, stiff ear cartilage)
- Genitals, male (scrotum flat and smooth in preterm → testes hang with deep ridges)
- Genitals, female (clitoris prominent in preterm → labia majora prominent in term)

Attachment behaviors: Initial assessment of maternal-infant bonding may begin with observation of maternal response to the infant after birth. Note response of other family members present. Continue observations whenever the infant interacts with mother, particularly during feedings, with the father, or with other family members.

Newborn nutrition is an essential measure to a successful transition, though the type of feeding is best decided in the antepartal period. Human milk is the preferred choice over formal prepared milk for the first year of life, due to the protective elements passed to the newborn. However, the nurse should support the mother in her choice of type of feeding.

The newborn is protected from injury through prophylactic eye treatment, vitamin K administration, and hepatitis B vaccine. The newborn is also given an initial screening for inborn errors of metabolism. The newborn may be classified as "high risk" according to birth weight, gestational age, or pathphysiological problems. Such a newborn may require intensive care with skilled nursing care and personnel with specialized knowledge.

NEWBORN ASSESSMENT

Skin

Skin integrity (absence of lesions, drainage, etc.), including the following:

- Color: **Pallor** (pale appearance) or **cyanosis** (bluish tinge) could indicate poor circulation or oxygenation; flushing could indicate increased blood flow to the skin due to infection; or **jaundice** (yellow tinge).

Nurse Alert The appearance of jaundice in the newborn prior to 24 hours of life is an indicator of an abnormally rapid rate of red blood cell destruction.

- Skin texture, dryness, or moisture (vervix caseosa is light on term newborn, heavy on premature infant, and scant to absent on post-term infant); temperature is generally above 36.5°C (97.7°F); note that sole creases should involve the heel.
- **Blanching/capillary refill** (pallor followed by return of flush after pressure; less than 3 seconds indicates circulatory adequacy).
- Birth marks or other skin color deviations (non-pathologic) may be noted.
- **Ecchymosis** (blue/black areas or bruises often from trauma) or abrasions (indicating scraping trauma), or **petechiae**, small pinpoint hemorrhages, could indicate a bleeding disorder due to lack of platelets.

Hair

- Note color, distribution, quality, texture, and elasticity. The newborn may have minimal hair on its head or a copious amount, particularly if post-term. Cultural variations in coarseness or curliness of hair may be noted, but hair and scalp should be clean and without lesions.
- Lanugo (fine hair) may be noted on the upper back. Unusual hair distribution on the face, arms, trunk, or legs could indicate pathology.
- Balding in an infant could suggest a need for more frequent position changes for sleep.
- Inspect the scalp for edema or hematoma or flaky skin, which could indicate caput succedaneum, cephalhematoma, scalp irritation, or infection.

Fingers

- Cyanotic fingertips may indicate respiratory or cardiac dysfunction.
- Nails should be smooth and flexible.

Head and Neck

- Size, shape, and symmetry: Monitor increasing head size; report extreme asymmetry for further evaluation.
- Fontanels are open resulting in soft area: Note bulging, which could indicate increased intracranial pressure or a depression/sinking in the fontanel area which could indicate dehydration.
- Note swollen neck glands, neck stiffness, or decreased range of motion.
- Report any shift in the trachea (possible lung problem), or mass in the neck.

Eyes and Vision

- Note the size, symmetry, color, and movement of the eyes, as well as exterior structures and spacing between the eyes; report deviations from expected straight palpebral fissures (upward slant normally noted in Asian

clients). Down syndrome may be characterized by epicanthal folds, upward palpebral slant, and **hypertelorism** (large spacing between eyes).
- Eyelids should be smooth without drooping or malposition; note blink reflex.
- Examine pupils for roundness, equal size, reactivity to light, accommodation, and size, color, and clarity of the iris (black and white speckling is seen in Down syndrome).
- The lens of the eye is normally not visible; white or gray spots could indicate cataracts.
- The newborn will have periods of alertness during which faces and bright objects will elicit staring and following of the object or face with the eyes.
- Report: Unusual eye movement, strabismus (may be normal in newborns), or excessively crossed eyes.

Ears and Hearing
- Inspect external ear structures for alignment; note flexibility of ear cartilage.
- Infant should respond to loud noise (startle reflex).

Mouth, Throat, Nose, Sinuses, and Neck
- Monitor oral area for intact palate (note cleft in lip or palate).
- Report any flaring of the nostrils, which could indicate respiratory distress.
- Note lesions of throat, mouth, or lips, and redness or drainage indicating infection.
- Fissures, stomatitis, or glossitis may indicate fluid and nutritional deficits.
- White patches in infants may indicate candidiasis.
- Palpate the head and neck for lymph nodes and report swollen, tender, or warm nodes that may indicate the presence of infection.

Chest
Heart, Neck Vessels, Pulses, and Blood Pressure
- Chest shape, symmetry, and movement should be noted. Report significant retraction of chest muscles, which could indicate respiratory distress.
- Assess nipples for symmetry.
- Listen to the heart with the infant in a supine position; note heart murmurs and record the location and volume intensity.
- Note indications of congenital heart disease (i.e., difficulty breathing, frothy sputum).
- Neck vein distention could indicate congestive heart failure.
- Report if infant becomes fatigued or short of breath during feeding as these are signs of decreased circulation or cardiac function.

- Resting pulse range for newborns is 110 to 160 beats per minute with slight irregularity. Count for a full minute.
- Blood pressure may not be assessed in a healthy newborn, except with internal monitoring in critical care. Newborn blood pressure may be 70–50/30–45 mm Hg.

Lungs and Respiration

- Breath sounds should be clear. Decreased or absent breath sounds could indicate lung congestion or consolidation.
- Abnormal breath sounds should be described instead of labeled to promote diagnosis and monitoring by various health-care providers.
- Respiratory rate range for newborns is 30 to 60 breaths per minute. Count for a full minute.

Abdomen

- Always auscultate before palpation or percussion of the abdomen to avoid altering current bowel sound pattern with artificial stimulation of bowel activity.
- Gently palpate the abdomen; *do not* palpate the abdomen if Wilms tumor is present.
- Examine all four quadrants of the abdomen: Cylindrical appearance without distension (gastrointestinal [GI] problem), or hollow appearance (possible diaphramatic hernia).
- Report visible peristaltic waves, which may indicate pathologic state.
- Note absence of or asymmetrical abdominal reflex.
- Note abdomen while newborn is crying, which increases intra-abdominal pressure, and inspect for hernia.
- Report hyperperistalsis indicated by hyperactive bowel sounds, or an absence of bowel sounds, both of which may indicate a GI disorder.
- Lack of tympany on percussion could indicate a full stomach or presence of fluid or solid tumor; avoid assessment of stomach immediately after feeding.
- Note guarding and tenderness, particularly rebound tenderness, or pain, which could indicate inflammation or infection.

Genitourinary

- Note urinary and genital structures, size, and appearance.
- Note and report: Undescended testes (cryptorchidism), urinary meatus that is not central at the tip of the shaft of the penis, large scrotal sac (possible hernia), or enlarged clitoris.

 Nurse Alert **Some conditions will produce a different genital appearance. Try not to react or show concern to parents.**

- If swelling, skin lesions, inflammation, drainage, or irregularities are noted, report for follow-up assessment for possible infection.
- Anal protrusions, hemorrhoids, lesions, irritation, or mucosal tags should be noted and may require follow-up.

Back and Extremities

- Note any lack of or difficulty in mobility, or overtly uneven limbs.
- With the newborn lying prone, note if curvature of the spine (possible **congenital scoliosis**) is present and report for further examination.
- Muscle weakness or paresis (may indicate neurologic problem or nutritional deficit), or extreme asymmetry of strength in extremities, hands, and fingers should be noted.

Many developmental delays are evident or detected during the newborn assessment. Examinations at 6 weeks and later with a developmental assessment tool, such as the Denver II or other inventory, should be monitored and deficits reported along with any relevant historical data. Assistance and referrals are provided to the family as needed.

CAPUT SUCCEDANEUM

WHAT WENT WRONG?

Caput succedaneum is a result of the birth trauma during a vertex presentation. Trauma results in serum and blood accumulation in the tissue over the suture lines of the scalp.

SIGNS AND SYMPTOMS

- Edematous tissue is noted over the suture lines of the scalp.
- The infant usually demonstrates no symptoms.

TEST RESULTS

No definitive test is required; the diagnosis is made on observational assessment.

TREATMENT

No specific treatment is necessary and the swelling resolves in a few days.

NURSING INTERVENTION

Reassure the mother and family that the swelling will subside and that the infant is not in pain.

CEPHALHEMATOMA

WHAT WENT WRONG?

Cephalhematoma occurs when the blood vessels are broken during labor and delivery and bleeding occurs between the bone and the periosteum.

SIGNS AND SYMPTOMS

The boundaries of the bleeding between the bones are sharply demarcated. The symptoms are usually not present at birth but develop within 24 to 48 hours.

TEST RESULTS

The diagnosis is made through observation.

TREATMENT

No treatment is indicated. The lesion normally resolves in 2 weeks to 1 or 2 months.

NURSING INTERVENTIONS

Affected newborns are at greater risk for jaundice and the nursing care is directed toward monitoring the newborn for jaundice and the effects of hyper-bilirubinemia.

HYDROCEPHALUS

WHAT WENT WRONG?

Hydrocephalus is a condition involving disruption of the circulation and absorption of cerebral spinal fluid (CSF), resulting in an accumulation of CSF in the ventricles of the brain (see Fig. 12.1). This condition causes the ventricles of the brain to dilate and increases intracranial pressure. There are two types of hydrocephalus:

- **Noncommunicating hydrocephalus:** Caused by an obstruction of CSF flow.
- **Communicating hydrocephalus:** Caused by disruption of CSF absorption.

SIGNS AND SYMPTOMS

- Rapidly increasing head circumference in infants
- Bulging and widening of fontanels in infants
- Underdeveloped neck muscles
- Shiny thin scalp
- Distended scalp veins
- Setting-sun sign where the sclera is above the iris
- Irritability

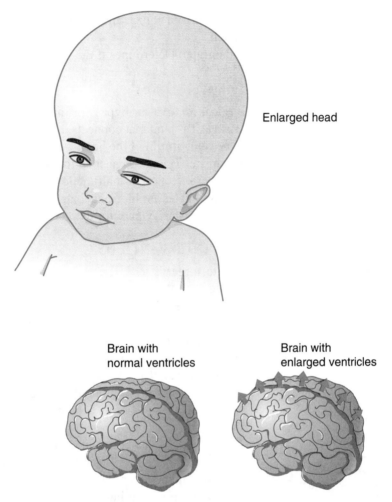

Enlarged head

Brain with
normal ventricles

Brain with
enlarged ventricles

Figure 12.1 • Ventricles of the brain: normal and enlarged

- Projectile vomiting
- Shrill cry
- Anorexia
- Weak sucking
- Nuchal rigidity
- Arnold-Chiari malformation

TEST RESULTS

- Head circumference measurement to detect enlargement
- CT scan: Visualizes the ventricles to determine if the ventricles are dilated

- MRI scan: Visualizes the ventricles to determine if the ventricles are dilated
- Radiograph: Determines if the skull is thinning or widening

TREATMENTS

- Surgical removal or bypass of the obstruction using a ventriculoperitoneal (VP) shunt that connects the ventricles to the peritoneal cavity or to the right atrium of the heart.
- Administer Tylenol as needed for postoperative pain.
- VP shunt infection or malfunction:
  - Administer antibiotic such as Vancomycin IV.
  - Administer Tylenol for temperature that is >101.3°F (38.5°C).

NURSING INTERVENTIONS

- Prior to surgery:
  - Measure the head circumference daily and report increases of 0.5 cm to the primary health-care provider.
  - Monitor for increased intracranial pressure.
  - Monitor vital signs every 4 hours.
  - Strict intake and output measurement.
  - Provide small feedings due to the risk of vomiting.
  - Burp the newborn frequently during feedings.
  - Support the newborn's head during feedings.
- After surgery:
  - Position the newborn flat on the non-operative side to prevent the cerebral spinal fluid from rapidly draining.
  - Assess the level of consciousness.
  - Monitor for vomiting.
  - Assess for infection and VP shut malfunction:
    - Severe headaches
    - Irritability
    - Vomiting
    - Redness along the shunt
    - Fluid around the VP shunt valve
    - Fever
    - Lethargy
  - Assess for abdominal distention resulting from paralytic ileus due to the VP shunt.
  - Explain the disorder and treatment to the family and explain that the VP shunt may have to be replaced periodically to accommodate the infant's growth. Also explain how to identify infection or malfunctioning of the VP shunt, and to call the health-care provider immediately if it should occur.

HYPERBILIRUBINEMIA

WHAT WENT WRONG?

Hyperbilirubinemia is an excessive level of bilirubin in the blood. Bilirubin is an end product from the breakdown of red blood cells that results in a jaundice appearance of the skin. Jaundice is classified as physiologic and pathologic. Physiologic jaundice is considered normal and becomes visible when the serum bilirubin reaches 5 to 7 mg/dL; the bilirubin levels begin to fall after the fourth day of life and returns to an adult stability in about 14 days.

SIGNS AND SYMPTOMS

It is important to differentiate physiologic jaundice from pathologic jaundice, which must be treated as a disease entity. Pathologic jaundice occurs in the first 24 hours after birth and is a result of excessive destruction of red blood cells.

TEST RESULTS

In pathological jaundice the total serum bilirubin is higher than 12 mg/dL in full-term infants and higher than 15 mg/dL in preterm infants.

TREATMENTS

- ◐ Prevent bilirubin encephalopathy.
- ◐ Phototherapy.
- ◐ Exchange transfusions are necessary if phototherapy does not alleviate the excessively high bilirubin levels quickly enough.

NURSING INTERVENTIONS

- ◐ When the newborn is placed under phototherapy, the majority of all skin surfaces should be exposed and the position changed frequently.
- ◐ Protect the eyes of the newborn from the fluorescent light with eye shields that are properly sized and positioned to cover the eyes completely.

 Nurse Alert **The infant's eyes should be closed before the shields are applied so that the risk of cornea damage from the eye dressing is eliminated.**

NEONATAL HYPOGLYCEMIA

WHAT WENT WRONG?

Transient neonatal hypoglycemia occurs when the newborn's blood glucose concentration is lower than 45 mg/dL in healthy full-term newborns, and lower than 36 mg/dL in newborns that are born at risk for illness or are premature.

TEST RESULTS

- Direct analysis of the blood glucose concentration is necessary to accurately confirm the diagnosis.
- Destrostix or Chemstrips can be used to estimate the blood glucose levels but the most accurate test is done in the laboratory.

TREATMENTS

- Provide the first feeding early after birth to maintain normoglycemia and prevent hypoglycemia.
- Oral glucose feeding can be used; however, human or formula milk is just as effective.
- Intravenous glucose is used when feeding is not effective.

NURSING INTERVENTIONS

- Monitor for signs and symptoms of hypoglycemia in the newborn.
- Institute measures to minimize the risk of hypoglycemia:
  - Reduce environmental stressors that predispose the newborn to blood glucose deficiency such as:
    - Cold stress
    - Prolonged feeding times
    - Increased respiratory efforts
  - When oral feedings are ineffective, intravenous glucose infusions are required.
- Protect the newborn from the side effects of hypertonic solution, such as circulatory overload and intracellular dehydration.

HYPERGLYCEMIA

WHAT WENT WRONG?

Hyperglycemia is defined as a blood glucose concentration greater than 125 mg/dL in full-term infants, and greater than 150 mg/dL in preterm infants.

SIGNS AND SYMPTOMS

- Hyperglycemia is usually asymptomatic.
- It is most often detected on a routine screening.

TEST RESULTS

- Destrostix or Chemstrips can reveal blood glucose levels.
- Serum glucose performed in the laboratory is most accurate.

TREATMENTS

- The initial treatment is the reduction of glucose intake.
- If dietary control is ineffective, low-dose infusion of insulin may be administered.

NURSING INTERVENTIONS

- ◐ Glucose levels are monitored very frequently.
- ◐ Numerous heel sticks are required; the nurse should be careful to rotate the sites to avoid tissue damage.

GALACTOSEMIA

WHAT WENT WRONG?

Galactosemia is a rare inborn error of carbohydrate metabolism resulting in the newborn's inability to convert galactose to glucose, which results in toxicity to tissues in the brain, kidneys, and nervous system.

SIGNS AND SYMPTOMS

- ◐ Vomiting and diarrhea are common symptoms.
- ◐ The infant becomes jaundiced by the second week of life.
- ◐ Cataracts are detectable by 2 months of age.
- ◐ The newborn is also lethargic and hypotonic.

TEST RESULTS

- ◐ The diagnosis is made on the basis of the infant's physical assessment history.
- ◐ Newborn screening for the disease is mandated in many states.
- ◐ Laboratory studies reveal decreased levels of galactose in the blood and galactose transferase activity in the erythrocytes.

TREATMENTS

- ◐ Treatment includes eliminating all milk and lactose-containing foods from the newborn's diet, including breast milk.
- ◐ Newborns are supplemented with soy-based formula.

NURSING INTERVENTIONS

- ◐ Teach the family about the nutritional intake and dietary restrictions.
- ◐ The nurse should incorporate the registered dietitian regimen in her plan of care for the newborn.
- ◐ Teach the family to read nutrition labels; maintaining dietary restrictions is essential.

MAPLE SYRUP URINE DISEASE

WHAT WENT WRONG?

5 In maple syrup urine disease the branched-chain amino acids are defective or absent due to a genetic disorder, resulting in an increase in branched-chain amino acids and ketoacids (byproducts) causing a burnt sugar smell in the urine.

SIGNS AND SYMPTOMS

- ◐ Maple syrup odor from urine
- ◐ Seizures
- ◐ Difficulty feeding
- ◐ Moro reflex absent
- ◐ Abnormal respirations

TEST RESULTS

- ◐ Serum: Increased branched-chain amino acids
- ◐ Urine: Increased branched-chain amino acids
- ◐ Blood gases: Acidosis

TREATMENTS

- ◐ Increase dietary thiamine.
- ◐ Avoid dietary isoleucine, valine, and leucine.
- ◐ Hemodialysis to remove branched-chain amino acids from the body.

NURSING INTERVENTIONS

- ◐ Perform urine and blood tests following the first day of feeding.
- ◐ Assess diapers for maple syrup odor.
- ◐ Teach parents the importance of avoiding foods that contain isoleucine, valine, and leucine.

PHENYLKETONURIA (PKU)

WHAT WENT WRONG?

5 Phenylketonuria is a genetic disorder that occurs because of a dysfunctional phenylalanine hydroxylase enzyme that is used to convert phenylalanine to tyrosine, resulting in accumulation of phenylalanine in the body that can cause mental retardation.

Nurse Alert The child has normal blood phenylalanine levels at birth; however, levels increase after birth and can result in irreversible damage by 2 years of age if not detected and treated.

SIGNS AND SYMPTOMS

- ◐ Family history of phenylketonuria
- ◐ Mental retardation as early as 4 months of age
- ◐ Dry skin
- ◐ Macrocephaly

- Irritable
- Hyperactive
- Musty skin odor
- Seizures (later years)

TEST RESULTS

- Guthrie Screening Test: Increased phenylalanine level in blood 4 days after birth
- Chromatography: Increased phenylalanine level in blood 4 days after birth

TREATMENTS

- Maintain blood levels of phenylalanine between 3 mg/dL and 9 mg/dL by restricting dietary phenylalanine (protein-rich foods).
- Administer enzymatic hydrolysate of casein (lofenalac, pregestimil) in place of milk.

NURSING INTERVENTIONS

- 5 Explain to the family that the child should avoid eggs, meat, fish, poultry, breads, aspartame, and cheese for the child's entire life.
- The phenylalanine level in the blood must be tested throughout the child's life to ensure that phenylalanine remains within the desired levels.

Nurse Alert **Be alert for signs of phenylalanine deficiency (anorexia, skin rashes, anemia, diarrhea, lethargy) that might occur as a result of too little phenylalanine in the diet.**

RESPIRATORY DISTRESS SYNDROME

WHAT WENT WRONG?

Premature infants born at less than 36 weeks gestation may develop respiratory distress syndrome or hyaline membrane disease (HMD) due to a lack of surfactant to keep the alveoli open.

SIGNS AND SYMPTOMS

- Breathing greater than 60 breath per minute
- Retractions (suprasternal and substernal)
- Grunting
- Nasal flaring
- Cyanosis
- Flaccid

TEST RESULTS

◐ Diagnosis is based on the infant's history, physical examination, lab results, and chest x-rays.

◐ Chest x-ray reveals fibrosis of the lungs.

TREATMENTS

◐ Prenatal steroids

◐ Administration of exogenous surfactant

◐ Diuretics

◐ Bronchodilators

◐ Oxygen therapy

③ NURSING INTERVENTIONS

◐ Ongoing physical examinations.

◐ Assess the infant's response to respiratory therapy.

◐ Monitor pulse oximetry and arterial oxygen concentration.

◐ Hyperventilation and suctioning when indicated.

 Nurse Alert **Watch oxygen levels closely because there is controversy regarding benefit versus detriment from oxygen therapy. Excessive oxygen can result in mortality or morbidity including retinal damage, bronchopulmonary dysplasia, nerve damage, or growth disturbance.**

HIRSCHSPRUNG DISEASE

WHAT WENT WRONG?

⑤ Hirschsprung disease is a congenital condition where there is a lack of nerve cells in the colon, causing a lack of peristalsis that results in stool being unable to be pushed through the colon.

 Nurse Alert **Hirschsprung disease is common in Down syndrome.**

SIGNS AND SYMPTOMS

◐ ⑤ Failure to pass stool (meconium) within the first 48 hours following birth

◐ Abdominal distention

◐ Abdominal mass

◐ Ribbon-like or liquid stool

◐ Sunken eyes

- ○ Pallor
- ○ Dehydration
- ○ Irritable
- ○ Weight loss
- ○ Lethargic

Nurse Alert **Monitor for fecal vomiting or bile stained vomitus as peristalsis may reverse and propel feces upward and out of the mouth.**

TEST RESULTS

- ○ Abdominal x-ray: Shows distended areas of the small and large intestines with little stool in the lower intestine near the anus.
- ○ Rectal biopsy: Absence of nerve ganglion cells in the colon.
- ○ Full-thickness surgical biopsy: Absence of nerve ganglion cells in the colon.
- ○ Suction aspiration of rectum: Absence of nerve ganglion cells in the colon.
- ○ Anorectal manometry: Absence of nerve reflexes.
- ○ Barium enema: Examination of the large intestines shows strictures/narrowed areas, or intestinal obstructions (blockages), and dilated intestine above the blockage.

TREATMENTS

- ○ Supportive care to support nutritional intake with temporary ostomy.
- ○ Surgery: After 9 months of age—the affected portion of the colon is removed.

Nurse Alert **If the colon is obstructed, a temporary colostomy or ileostomy is performed to decompress the colon. Once decompressed, a second surgery is performed to remove the affected portion of the colon and remove the colostomy or ileostomy.**

NURSING INTERVENTIONS

- ○ Preoperatively:
  - • Nothing by mouth.
  - • Administer IV fluids as ordered to maintain fluid and electrolyte balance.
  - • Insert a nasogastric (NG) tube to decompress the upper GI tract.
  - • Administer normal saline or mineral oil enemas to clean the bowel.
  - • Administer antibiotics as ordered.

◑ Postoperatively:
- Strict input and output measurement to monitor fluid levels closely.
- Provide care for the colostomy or ileostomy, if necessary.
- Monitor bowel sounds.
- Begin feeding by mouth when bowel sounds are present.
- Nothing should be placed in the rectum.
- Monitor for constipation.

◑ Explain the disorder and treatment to the family and instruct them on the proper care for the wound and how to care for the colostomy or ileostomy, if necessary. Tell the family to call the health-care provider at the first signs of constipation, dehydration, fever, vomiting, or diarrhea.

Nurse Alert **Don't use tap water in the enema since this can induce water intoxication. Return of anal sphincter control and complete continence can take months to develop.**

CONGENITAL HEART CONDITIONS

Fetal circulation involves the blood moving from the right side of the heart to the left side while bypassing the lungs. Openings were in place between the right and left atria and the right and left ventricles to facilitate the blood flow. (See Chapter 7) When the newborn enters the extrauterine environment the pressures change in the chest, causing the lungs to open, and the cardiac blood flow changes. The openings in the heart usually close, leaving only the valves and pressures to promote blood flow through the heart and lungs.

WHAT WENT WRONG?

Occasionally the openings in the heart remain intact after the lungs are functional. These openings/defects may result in a shunting of blood from right to left heart without oxygenation from the lungs, or from left to right ventricles causing recirculation of oxygenated blood through the lungs with a decrease of blood moving to the body. The decreased circulation to the body, or circulation of deoxygenated blood to tissues, results in poorly perfused and poorly oxygenated newborn tissues and newborn distress. The degree of newborn distress resulting from a defect or combination of defects depends on the impact the defect has on tissue perfusion or oxygenation.

SIGNS AND SYMPTOMS

Varied based on defect (see specific defect).

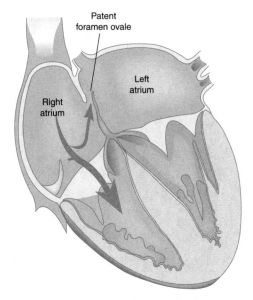

Figure 12.2 • Anatomy of the fetal heart (inside view).

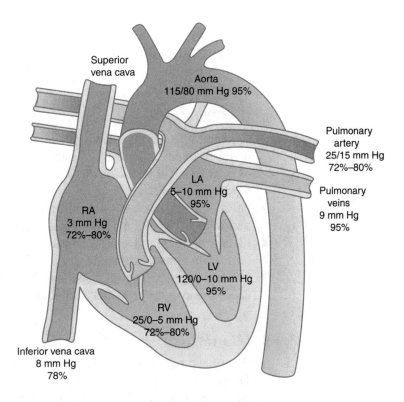

Figure 12.3 • Adult heart structures and pressures.

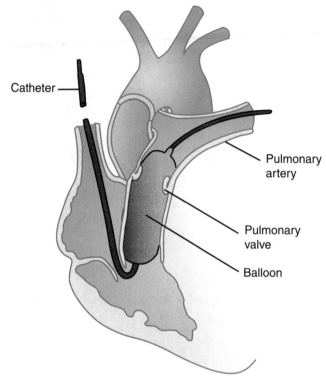

Figure 12.4 • Cardiac catheterization.

② TEST RESULTS

- Cardiac catheterization: Catheters are inserted into the heart via a large peripheral vein and advanced into the heart to measure pressures and oxygen levels in the heart chambers and visualize heart structures and blood flow patterns
- Pulse oximetry (Spo_2): A device used to evaluate the degree of oxygen saturation in the blood using a small infrared light probe.
- Electrocardiogram: Detects electrical events, and normal and abnormal cardiac rhythms in the heart.
- Echocardiogram: Two-dimensional Doppler evaluation to detect evidence of valve leakage, and cardiac anatomy, size, and function.

⑤ TREATMENTS

- Open-heart repair with cardiopulmonary bypass.
- Treatment of choice is surgical patch closure.
- Atrial septal defect (ASD) may require mitral valve replacement.

NURSING INTERVENTIONS FOR CARDIAC CATHETERIZATION

- Prepare the patient for cardiac catheterization:
  - Take complete nursing history.
  - Patient must have nothing by mouth for 4 to 6 hours.
  - Perform a complete assessment including calculation of body surface area.
  - Check for allergies: Allergies to iodine, contrast dyes, and shellfish should be relayed to the physician prior to the procedure.
  - Document baseline assessment of pedal pulses and pulse oximetry.
  - Utilize child life specialists to alleviate anxiety for the family.
  - Explain specific aspects of the procedure such as the placement of the IV and electrocardiogram (ECG) electrodes.
  - Demonstrate how the skin will be washed with brown soap and how the skin will be numbed.
  - Explain how the contrast affects the patient, and how sedation will make the infant respond, emphasizing that the newborn should have no discomfort.
- Care of the patient post–cardiac catheterization:
  - Monitor the patient with a cardiac monitor and pulse oximeter prior to discharge.
  - Take vital signs every 15 minutes for the first hour, and hourly thereafter.
  - Monitor the patient for the following:
    - Temperature and color distal to the catheter insertion site
    - A pulse of the extremity distal to the catheter insertion site
  - Monitor for trends and assess for possible hypotension, tachycardia, and bradycardia.
  - Check the pressure dressing for evidence of bleeding.
  - Observe for bleeding at the insertion site or evidence of hematoma.
  - Monitor intake and output for diuresis from contrast material.
  - The family should be provided with education upon discharge to:
    - Observe the site for signs of inflammation and infection.
    - Monitor for fever.
    - Avoid strenuous activities for a few days.
    - Avoid tub baths for 48 to 72 hours.
    - Use acetaminophen or ibuprofen for discomfort.

Nurse Alert **If bleeding occurs, apply direct continuous pressure 1 inch above the percutaneous skin site; this will localize pressure over the vessel puncture.**

Nurse Alert **It is important for the nurse to assess for latex allergies prior to catheterization. Some catheters used in the catheterization laboratory have latex balloons. If the newborn has a latex allergy, the balloon can precipitate a life-threatening reaction.**

NURSING INTERVENTIONS FOR NEWBORN UNDERGOING CARDIAC SURGERY

○ Provide preoperative care for the newborn as follows:
- Make inquiries to parents and caregivers as to any questions they may have about the procedure.
- Orient the family to strange surroundings prior to surgery day.
- Check chart for signed informed consent forms.
- Check identification band with surgical personnel to ensure identity.
- Ensure that side rails are securely fastened.
- Use restraints for transport.
- Check laboratory values for signs of systemic alterations.
- Bathe and groom the newborn.
- Provide mouth care for comfort while npo.
- Cleanse operative site with prescribed method.
- Administer antibiotics as ordered.
- Remove jewelry, makeup, prosthetic.
- Check for loose teeth.
- Institute preoperative teaching to reduce anxiety.
- Prepare the family for postoperative procedures such as insertion of a nasogastric tube, wound care, and use of a monitoring apparatus.
- Administer preoperative sedation.

○ Provide postoperative care for the newborn as follows:
- Make sure the newborn is in a safe position of comfort according to the physician's order.
- Perform stat orders.
- Use proper hand washing.
- Assess the wound for bleeding and signs of infection.
- Provide appropriate wound care.
- Assess breath sounds.
- Perform neurologic checks.
- Take frequent vital signs.
- Administer fluids to prevent hypotension.
- Monitor fluid losses through the chest tube.
- Administer pharmacologic support as ordered.
- Monitor electrolytes and supplement with infusion as ordered.
- Administer sedatives and analgesics for comfort.

- Allow caregivers to visit as soon as possible.
- Explain procedures and equipment to caregivers.
- Encourage caregivers to ask questions.
- **4** Involve child life specialist and social services in the care to support the child and family.

ATRIAL SEPTAL DEFECT (ASD)

WHAT WENT WRONG?

ASD is an abnormal opening between the atria that allows blood to flow from the left atrium into the right atrium. Left atrium pressure is slightly higher, which allows blood to flow from the left to the right atrium. This abnormal blood flow causes the following:

- Increase of oxygenated blood into the right atrium
- Right atrium and right ventricle enlargement

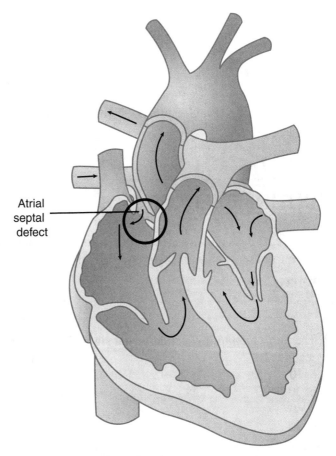

Atrial septal defect

Figure 12.5 • Atrial septal defect (ASD).

SIGNS AND SYMPTOMS

- ◐ Patients are sometimes asymptomatic.
- ◐ ASD may precipitate congestive heart failure.
- ◐ A murmur characteristic of ASD is heard on auscultation.
- ◐ Increased pulmonary blood flow may lead to pulmonary vascular obstruction or emboli.

TEST RESULTS

- ◐ Cardiac catheterization: Reveals septal defect and any structural changes or defects.
- ◐ Pulse oximetry (Spo_2): Oxygen level may be within normal range.
- ◐ Electrocardiogram: Atrial septal defect is noted with right ventricular hypertrophy.
- ◐ Echocardiogram: Septal defect and ventricular hypertrophy are evident.

TREATMENT

- ◐ ASD may require mitral valve replacement.

NURSING INTERVENTIONS

- ◐ Provide care for the patient during cardiac catheterization.
- ◐ Provide preoperative and postoperative care (see above).

✔ ROUTINE CHECKUP 1

1. Beverly, 3 days old, is scheduled for a cardiac catheterization. What approach should the nurse use when teaching preoperatively?

Answer:

2. The nurse monitoring a child's vital signs should count the heart rate for how many seconds?
   a. 10
   b. 30
   c. 60
   d. 90

Answer:

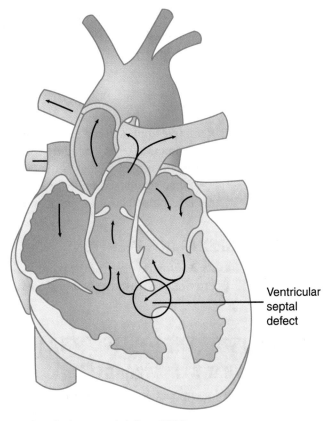

Figure 12.6 • Ventricular septal defect (VSD).

VENTRICULAR SEPTAL DEFECT (VSD)

WHAT WENT WRONG?

VSD is an abnormal opening causing complications between the right and left ventricles. The defect may vary in size from a pinhole to the actual absence of the septum.

SIGNS AND SYMPTOMS

- Blood flows from the left ventricle into the pulmonary artery.
- Increased pulmonary blood flow and increased pulmonary resistance.
- Congestive heart failure.

TEST RESULTS

- Cardiac catheterization: Ventricular defects and cardiomegaly will be evident.

- Pulse oximetry (SpO$_2$): Oxygen saturation will be decreased.
- Electrocardiogram: Signs of cardiomegaly noted.
- Echocardiogram: Septal defect, cardiomegaly, and altered cardiac function noted.

4,5 TREATMENTS

- Palliative approach includes the following:
  - Pulmonary artery banding (band around the pulmonary artery)
- Complete surgical repair is the treatment of choice:
  - Purse string technique for small defects
  - Dacron patch for larger openings

NURSING INTERVENTIONS

- 4,5 Provide care for the patient during cardiac catheterization.
- Provide preoperative and postoperative care (see above).

PATENT DUCTUS ARTERIOSUS (PDA)

WHAT WENT WRONG?

1 Patent ductus arteriosus occurs when the artery connecting the aorta and the pulmonary artery in fetal circulation fails to close during the first few weeks of life. The continued patency allows blood from the aorta to flow back to the pulmonary artery, resulting in a left-to-right shunt. This altered circulation causes the following:

- Increased workload on the left side of the heart
- Pulmonary congestion and resistance
- Right ventricular hypertrophy

2 SIGNS AND SYMPTOMS

- Patient may be asymptomatic.
- Characteristics of congestive heart failure.

2 TEST RESULTS

- Cardiac catheterization: Patent ductus and right ventricular hypertrophy evident
- Pulse oximetry (SpO$_2$): Oxygen saturation decreased
- Electrocardiogram: Signs of ventricular hypertrophy noted
- Echocardiogram: Septal defects and ventricular hypertrophy noted

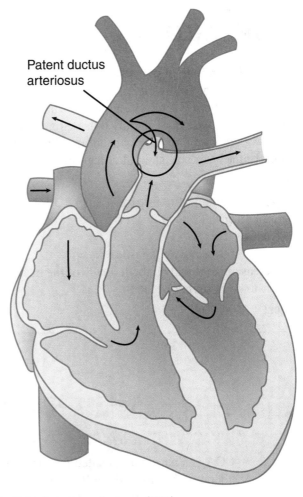

Patent ductus
arteriosus

Figure 12.7 • Patent ductus arteriosus (PDA).

4.5 TREATMENTS

Palliative approach includes the following:

- Administration of indomethacin (prostaglandin inhibitor)
- Application of coils to occlude the PDA

Surgical treatment:

- Ligation and clipping of the patent vessel

NURSING INTERVENTIONS

- 4.5 Provide care for the patient during cardiac catheterization.
- Provide preoperative and postoperative care (see above).

✔ ROUTINE CHECKUP 2

1. A chest echocardiogram will be ordered for the newborn with congenital heart disease to do which of the following?
   a. Display the bones of the chest and coloring of the cardiac structures
   b. Evaluate the vascular anatomy outside of the heart
   c. Show a graph of the electrical activity of the heart
   d. Determine heart size and pulmonary blood flow patterns

Answer:

2. Surgery for patent ductus arteriosus (PDA) prevents which of the following complications?
   a. Cyanosis
   b. Pulmonary vascular congestion
   c. Decreased workload on the left side of the heart
   d. Left-to-right shunt of blood

Answer:

COARCTATION OF THE AORTA (COA)

WHAT WENT WRONG?

COA is a narrowing located near the insertion of the ductus arteriosus. This alteration results in the following:

- Increased pressure in the head and neck area
- Decreased pressure distal to the obstruction in the body and lower extremities

➋ SIGNS AND SYMPTOMS

- High blood pressure and bounding pulses in the upper extremities.
- Lower extremities are cool with decreased pulses and blood pressure.
- Symptoms of congestive heart failure.
- Hypertension.

➋ TEST RESULTS

- Cardiac catheterization: Reveals the location of the aortic narrowing and VSD or PDA if present.
- Pulse oximetry (SpO_2): May be normal or decreased if CHF is present.

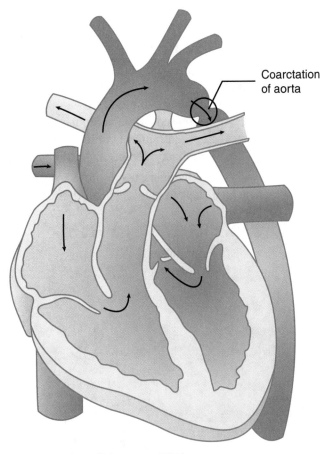

Figure 12.8 • Coarctation of the aorta (COA)

◐ Electrocardiogram: Signs of right and left ventricular hypertrophy are noted.
◐ Echocardiogram: Two-dimensional Doppler evaluation to detect evidence of valve leakage, and cardiac anatomy, size, and function.

4,5 TREATMENTS

◐ Balloon angioplasty
◐ Resection of the coarcted portion with end-to-end anastomosis of the aorta
◐ Enlargement of the constricted section by a graft prosthetic

NURSING INTERVENTIONS

◐ 4,5 Provide care for the patient during cardiac catheterization.
◐ Provide preoperative and postoperative care (see above).

AORTIC STENOSIS (AS)

WHAT WENT WRONG?

AS is a narrowing or a stricture of the aortic valve that results in the following:

- Resistance to blood flow in the left ventricle
- Decreased cardiac output
- Left ventricular hypertrophy
- Pulmonary venous and pulmonary arterial hypertension

1 The hallmark result of AS is hypertrophy of the left ventricular wall, which leads to increased end-diastolic pressure and pulmonary hypertension.

2 SIGNS AND SYMPTOMS

- Faint pulses
- Hypotension

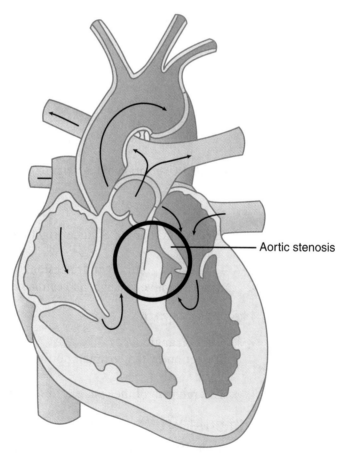

Aortic stenosis

Figure 12.9 • Aortic stenosis (AS).

- Tachycardia
- Poor feeding
- Exercise intolerance
- Chest pain
- Dizziness
- Characteristic murmur

2. TEST RESULTS

- Cardiac catheterization: Reveals septal defect and left ventricular hypertrophy
- Pulse oximetry (SpO_2): Decreased oxygen saturation levels
- Electrocardiogram: Evidence of ventricular hypertrophy
- Echocardiogram: Reveals aortic stenosis and any other cardiac defects

4,5 TREATMENTS

- Balloon angioplasty to provide blood flow
- Excision of a membrane
- Cutting of the fibromuscular ring

NURSING INTERVENTIONS

- 4,5 Provide care for the patient during cardiac catheterization.
- Provide preoperative and postoperative care (see above).

TETRALOGY OF FALLOT (TOF)

WHAT WENT WRONG?

The classic form of TOF has four defects:
- Ventricular septal defect
- Pulmonic stenosis
- Overriding aorta
- Right ventricular hypertrophy

2. SIGNS AND SYMPTOMS

- Cyanosis
- Hypoxia
- Anoxic spells when infant's oxygen supply exceeds blood supply (crying)

2. TEST RESULTS

- Cardiac catheterization: Reveals the four defects.
- Pulse oximetry (SpO_2): Decreased according to degree of deoxygenation.

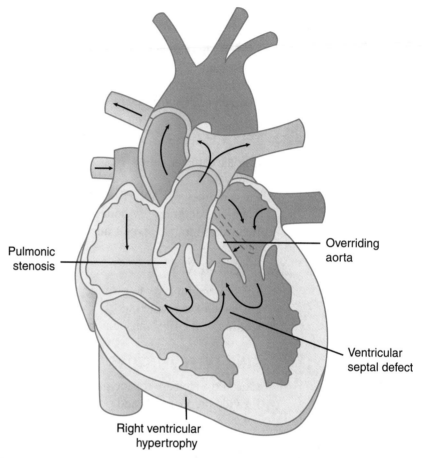

Figure 12.10 • Tetralogy of Fallot (TOF).

- Electrocardiogram: Signs of right ventricular hypertrophy are noted.
- Echocardiogram: The four defects are revealed.

TREATMENTS

- Blalock-Taussig procedure to increase pulmonary blood flow
- Complete repair by:
  - Closing the VSD
  - Resection of the infundibular stenosis
  - Enlarging the right ventricular outflow tract

NURSING INTERVENTIONS

- Provide care for the patient during cardiac catheterization.
- Provide preoperative and postoperative care (see above).

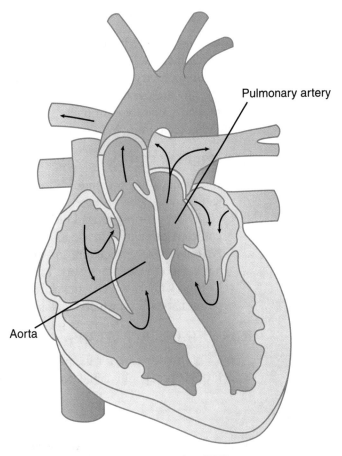

Figure 12.11 • Transposition of great arteries (TGA)

TRANSPOSITION OF GREAT ARTERIES (TGA)

WHAT WENT WRONG?

In transposition of great arteries, the pulmonary artery rises from the left ventricle and the aorta exits from the right ventricle.

- There is no communication between the systemic and pulmonary circulation.
- Life is sustained due to defects associated with the TGA.
- The common defects are patent ductus arteriosus and ventricular septal defect.

SIGNS AND SYMPTOMS

- Severely cyanotic
- Characteristics of congestive heart failure

🔑 TEST RESULTS

- Cardiac catheterization: Reveals vessel transposition, septal defects, and cardiomegaly.
- Pulse oximetry (SpO_2): Oxygen saturation levels are low.
- Electrocardiogram: May be normal for the newborn and later show signs of ventricular hypertrophy.
- Echocardiogram: Will reveal vessel transposition and septal defects.

🔑 TREATMENTS

- Intravenous prostaglandin E to increase blood mixing so that oxygen saturation is 75% or better.
- Atrial septostomy (Rashkind procedure) is performed during cardiac catheterization to increase mixing and maintain cardiac output.
- Arterial switch procedure to connect the main artery to the proximal aorta and the ascending aorta to the proximal pulmonary artery.
- Coronary arteries are switched from the proximal aorta to the proximal pulmonary artery, which creates a new aorta.

NURSING INTERVENTIONS

- 🔑 Provide care for the patient during cardiac catheterization.
- Provide preoperative and postoperative care (see above).

CONCLUSION

As the newborn transitions to extrauterine life, the nurse must assist in stabilizing the infant. The nurse must also frequently assess the newborn and family to detect any problems that might already exist or may occur after birth.

- Immediate newborn care involves airway clearance and temperature stabilization.
- Initial assessments include Apgar assessment at 1 minute and 5 minutes after birth, reactivity, gestational age assessment using a tool to determine neuromuscular and physical maturity, and attachment behaviors that reveal bonding or lack thereof.
- Assessment should be performed using a systems approach beginning immediately after birth.
- Early bonding with the mother through skin-to-skin contact is beneficial for the mother and child and also promotes temperature stability.
- Nutrition decisions are frequently made prior to birth. Human milk is preferred.
- Prophylactic eye treatment, vitamin K, and hepatitis B vaccine may be administered.
- Screening for congenital conditions, including inborn errors of metabolism, is performed.

◑ Newborn assessment is performed using a head-to-toe approach:
- Skin: Note color for cyanosis or jaundice, lesions, or other injuries.
- Hair: Presence and degree of lanugo may indicate preterm, term, or post-term status.
- Fingers: Cyanosis could indicate respiratory or cardiac dysfunction.
- Head and neck: Note size, symmetry, and fontanels as well as neck glands and trachea.
- Eyes and eyelids: Size, shape, movement/blink, and space between the eyes.
- Ears and hearing: External ear structure could indicate age; note hearing.
- Mouth, nose, and throat: Note cleft in nose or palate; nasal flaring may indicate respiratory distress.
- Chest: Note retractions that may indicate respiratory distress, or heart rate, heart sounds, or neck vein distension that indicates heart disease or failure.
- Lungs: Breath sounds should be clear; respiratory rate 30 to 60 breaths per minute.
- Abdomen: Assess gently, do not palpate if Wilms tumor is present; note bowel sounds, distension, peristaltic waves, and signs of hernia.
- Genitourinary: Note urinary and genital structures (descended testes, anal protrusions, hemorrhoids, irritation, or lesions).
- Back and extremities: Muscle strength, paresis, spinal curvature.

◑ Multiple conditions could occur before or during birth that are discovered during the newborn examination and require initial and follow-up care:
- Caput succedaneum: Edematous tissue over scalp suture lines
- Cephalhematoma: Broken blood vessels
- Hydrocephalus: Increased head size due to accumulation of CSF
- Hyperbilirubinemia: Jaundice within the first 24 hours after birth

？ FINAL CHECKUP

1. What are common symptoms of galactosemia?
 a. Yellow skin coloring
 b. Sensitivity to light
 c. Hyperactivity and hypertonicity
 d. Increased appetite and constipation

2. What measures might a nurse use to reduce the risk of newborn hypoglycemia?
 a. Cool the room to slow metabolism.
 b. Space meals at least 6 hours apart.
 c. Begin breast-feeding early after birth.
 d. Infuse nasogastric feeding with saline.

3. **What is a true statement about hyperbilirubinemia?**
   a. A serum bilirubin of 2 mg/dL occurring at 20 hours of life is pathologic.
   b. A serum bilirubin of 4 mg/dL occurring at 24 hours of life is pathologic.
   c. A serum bilirubin of 8 mg/dL occurring at 36 hours of life is pathologic.
   d. A serum bilirubin of 13 mg/dL occurring at 16 hours of life is pathologic.

4. **If bleeding occurs after a cardiac catheterization what should be the nurse's initial action?**
   a. Apply heparin ointment to stimulate clotting at the puncture site.
   b. Administer an anticoagulant to free clotting factors.
   c. Put pressure on the skin area 1 inch above the insertion site.
   d. Calm the parents by explaining that bleeding is expected and will stop spontaneously.

5. **Ventricular septal defect has which of the following blood flow patterns?**
   a. Decreased pulmonary blood flow
   b. Increased pulmonary blood flow
   c. Decreased left atrial blood flow
   d. Increased right atrial blood flow

6. **The nurse reinforces the physician's explanation that surgery should be performed for patent ductus arteriosus (PDA) to prevent what complications?**
   a. Hypoxemia
   b. Right-to-left shunt of blood
   c. Decreased workload on the left side of the heart
   d. Pulmonary vascular congestion

7. **What defect results in obstruction to blood flow?**
   a. Atrial septal defect
   b. Tricuspid atresia
   c. Aortic stenosis
   d. Transposition of the great arteries

8. **Galactosemia has been diagnosed in a breast-fed newborn. The therapeutic management in this situation would include what action?**
   a. Instruct the mother to stop breast-feeding the newborn.
   b. Provide amino acids to the mother to alter the breast milk.
   c. Feed the newborn a lactose-containing formula instead.
   d. Give the appropriate enzyme along with breast milk.

9. **What would be an important nursing intervention for a term infant receiving phototherapy?**
   a. Using sunscreen to protect infant's skin
   b. Monitoring the infant closely for signs of dehydration
   c. Keeping child diapered to collect frequent stools
   d. Informing the mother why breast-feeding must be discontinued

10. **What is a main factor that is responsible for respiratory distress syndrome in newborns?**
    a. Immature bronchioles
    b. Absence of alveolar oxygenation
    c. Inadequate surfactant production
    d. Overdeveloped alveoli

References

Hockenberry MJ. (2007). *Wong's Nursing Care of Infants and Children.* 8th ed. Philadelphia: Mosby.

Ladewig P, London M, & Davidson M. (2009). *Contemporary Maternal-Newborn Nursing Care.* 7th ed. New York: Pearson Education.

McKinney E. (2009). *Maternal-Child Nursing.* 3rd ed. Philadelphia: Elsevier Saunders.

ANSWERS

Routine Checkup 1

1. Direct teaching to her parents providing an overview of the process and including an explanation that the infant should be sedated and will experience minimal discomfort.
2. c

Routine Checkup 2

1. d
2. b

Final Checkup

1. a	2. c	3. d	4. c	5. b
6. d	7. c	8. a	9. b	10. c

Final Exam

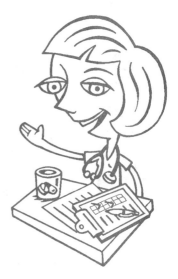

1. **What is an accurate description of a nurse whose primary role is to assess and plan the care for a new mother and perform teaching in preparing the child-bearing family for pregnancy?**
   a. Licensed practical nurse
   b. Registered nurse
   c. Certified nurse midwife
   d. Licensed vocational nurse

2. **What cultural religious ceremony could be accommodated without monitoring by the nurse?**
   a. Drinking of herbal teas by the client several times a day to restore balance
   b. Rubbing of a chemical ointment on the head and torso to drive away spirits
   c. Ingesting a pregnancy powder passed down from grandmother to mother to daughter
   d. Wearing a talisman to ward off pain and keep bad spirits away from the body

3. **Which example represents a cohabitation family?**
   a. Judy and her mother and father live in Kansas in the fall and Paris in the summer.
   b. Paula, age 20, and her boyfriend and their 2-year-old live in an apartment.
   c. Angela and her two fathers live in a house attached to her grandparents' home.
   d. a and b only.

4. **Sally says she lives with her mother, father, and brothers. Her family is probably classified as what type of family?**
   a. Reconstituted family
   b. Gay family
   c. Cohabited family
   d. Traditional family

5. The nurse tells Mr. Estavez, who wants to take his pregnant wife back to Spain for delivery, that the best care his wife can receive will be found in America. This is a possible example of what attitude?

    a. The need to bring in a translator

    b. Ethnocentric behavior

    c. Acculturated behavior

    d. Subcultural behavior

6. Nurses should be aware of what factors when assessing clients of a different ethnic or cultural group from their own?

    a. Effective methods of persuasion

    b. The nurses' personal bias

    c. Political views

    d. All the above

7. What factor should be considered first when a nurse assesses a pregnant client's growth and development?

    a. Relationship with husband

    b. Communication skills

    c. Religious preference

    d. Political party

8. A 21-year-old female client asks what would be the best type of birth control for her to use. The nurse assesses that the client currently smokes and has smoked since the age of 14. Which types of birth control method should the nurse avoid recommending?

    a. Oral contraceptives

    b. Depo-Provera injection

    c. Diaphragm

    d. Intrauterine device (IUD)

9. A 15-year-old female student presents to a high school nurse and states that she has not had her period in 4 weeks and does not know which at-home pregnancy test to purchase. Which type of test would be most accurate in determining if the student is pregnant?

    a. A test that can detect high levels of hCG

    b. A blood test at the health department

    c. A test that can detect high levels of testosterone

    d. A blood test for progesterone

10. Which nurse could serve as a primary care provider for a pregnant woman?

    a. Byron, who is a licensed practical nurse

    b. Briana, who is a registered nurse

    c. Jack, who is a certified nurse-midwife

    d. None of the above

11. **Family planning for an infertile couple should include what activities?**
    a. Discussing the adoption of a healthy baby
    b. Discussing contraception method options
    c. Providing care during menopause
    d. All of the above

12. **Mrs. Perkins visits the clinic for her second prenatal examination. What phase of pregnancy is she is in?**
    a. Puerperium phase
    b. Intrapartum phase
    c. Antipartum phase
    d. Postpartum phase

13. **What is a major reason the developmental stage of the expectant female could have an impact on a pregnancy?**
    a. None, really, the fetal developmental stage is more important.
    b. If the female is still living at home her mother can parent the newborn.
    c. The female who is an adolescent will have nutritional needs that may conflict with the needs of pregnancy.
    d. The older female has completed all of her developmental stages by the age of 40 and can focus more on the needs of a newborn.

14. **Clara, age 14 years, is admitted for dehydration secondary to continued vomiting in her first trimester of pregnancy. The nurse notes that she has her teddy bear and clings to her mother's arm. What would be the most likely explanation for Clara's behavior?**
    a. The stress of pregnancy has caused Clara to revert to a younger developmental stage.
    b. Clara's overprotective mother has spoiled Clara, which is why she is pregnant.
    c. The pregnancy has effected Clara's brain and caused her to become retarded.
    d. Clara is trying to deny that she is pregnant by acting like a baby herself.

15. **Betty, age 16 years, is pregnant and is admitted after experiencing hyperemesis gravidarum for the past 6 days. She is drowsy and speaks only when shaken or stimulated in some other way. What should the nurse keep in mind when assessing Betty?**
    a. Betty might have a fluid or electrolyte imbalance from the vomiting.
    b. Betty would be more responsive if her mother were not in the room.
    c. Betty's behavior is not important since her chief complaint is nausea and vomiting.
    d. Betty is an adolescent and may also be drowsy and sleepy when she is home.

16. **A nurse identifying high-risk obstetric clients would be most concerned about which expectant mother?**
    a. Andrea Petes, 3 months pregnant, who complained of foul smelling vaginal drainage last month
    b. Penelope Mund, 2 months pregnant, who cared for her niece as she recovered from appendicitis
    c. Carley Adrinde, 6 weeks pregnant, who has been nauseated the past 2 weeks and vomited daily
    d. Alley Bendera, who is 12 weeks pregnant and reports having breast tenderness and enlargement

17. **What category of growth and development focuses on weight and height?**
    a. Cognitive
    b. Physical
    c. Spiritual
    d. a and b

18. **Nancy is pregnant and asks what her "due" date should be. Her last menstrual period started on June 10, 2010. Using Nagele's rule, you calculate that her estimated date of delivery would be what date?**
    a. February 10, 2011
    b. February 17, 2011
    c. March 10, 2011
    d. March 17, 2011

19. **Sue is obese and is 2 months pregnant. What instructions should be provided in nutrition planning?**
    a. Eat a nutritious diet and gain about 15 to 20 pounds, depending on Sue's physical size.
    b. High intake of simple sugars is important to provide carbohydrates for fetal growth.
    c. If Sue is over the age of 40 she should eat low calories to avoid excess weight gain.
    d. Avoid foods such as organ meats and peanuts to prevent buildup of folic acid levels.

20. **What measure could be most effective in increasing the chances of obtaining pregnancy?**
    a. Douching before sex to clear debris that could block sperm.
    b. Having the male avoid sex or masturbation between attempted conception to increase sperm count.
    c. Ambulation after sex could mobilize sperm and move it to the ova.
    d. Exercise more than 10 hours each week to stimulate production and mobility of ova to the fallopian tubes.

21. **What information should be provided to a woman who has had a spontaneous abortion?**
    a. The fact that there is sometimes no distinct cause for miscarriage and no one is at fault.
    b. The gender of the fetus, so the parents can name the child and focus their grief.
    c. Grief should not be experienced since the woman can always get pregnant again.
    d. Methods for obtaining emergency contraception to avoid a repeat abortion.

22. **Testing for infertility would include what process?**
    a. Focusing on the partner who is most likely to blame.
    b. Begin testing if the couple is unable to conceive after trying a year.
    c. Performing testing if the couple can afford the option of in-vitro fertilization.
    d. Infertility focus should center on the older partner in the couple.

23. **What test for pregnancy would be most accurate?**
    a. A test that measured 60 mIU/mL hCG
    b. A test that measured 30 mIU/mL hCG
    c. A urine test done on a second voided specimen
    d. A urine test done after drinking gallons of fluid

24. **What period of pregnancy involves the completion of fetal organs and body parts?**
    a. Germinal period
    b. Fallopian period
    c. Fetal period
    d. Embryonic period

25. **Alecia is admitted to the hospital floor in active labor. She is in what phase of pregnancy?**
    a. Prenatal phase
    b. Intrapartal phase
    c. Antipartal phase
    d. Postpartum phase

26. **The prenatal phase of care for the woman and family would include what activities?**
    a. Discussing ways to promote delivering a healthy baby
    b. Discussing methods of contraception to prevent pregnancy
    c. Providing care during menopause to address the discomforts of hormones
    d. Administering pain medication for intermittent bleeding

27. **Trelina, 31 years old, is 4 months pregnant and has several small sores, sparse pubic hair, and a BMI of 62%. What is she most likely suffering from?**
    a. Scoliosis
    b. Cyanosis
    c. Malnutrition
    d. Depression

28. **July has low hematocrit and albumen levels as well as low serum levels of creatinine. What are the most probable implications of these symptoms?**
    a. Protein deficiency
    b. Renal damage
    c. Exposure to a toxic drug
    d. Vitamin B$_{12}$ anemia

29. **At the first prenatal visit the female, 36 years old, has bruised areas on her arms, a light skin color with no red or pink undertones, and swelling in her feet and legs. These symptoms can be described as what?**
    a. Edema, pallor, and delayed development
    b. Pallor, hypertelorism, and petechiae
    c. Edema, ecchymosis, and pallor
    d. None of the above

30. **What are behavioral style; and calm or lack of calm, relative to family members, aspects of?**
    a. Temperament
    b. Role designation
    c. Physique
    d. None the above

31. **Pectoriloquy is noted during the initial examination of a pregnant 23-year-old African-American female. What does she most likely suffer from?**
    a. Vaginal infection
    b. Lung consolidation
    c. Down syndrome
    d. Early contractions

32. **Stomatitis, glossitis, and fissures are symptoms common to disorders of what?**
    a. Ears and eyes
    b. Back and chest
    c. Skin and nails
    d. Mouth and tongue

33. **A client with condition Z, a recessive condition, feels guilty because she feels it is all her fault the baby may have condition Z. What would be the best response to the client?**
    a. "It is not your fault you have this gene; your child will get accustomed to it."
    b. "It is your genes that will cause the child to have the conditions but you could not control that."
    c. "Because condition Z is recessive, both you and the father would have to carry and pass on the gene in order for the child to have the condition."
    d. "Because condition Z is recessive, your gene has overpowered the gene of the father and caused the child to have the condition, but you shouldn't feel guilty."

34. **Sickle cell anemia is transmitted to a child through what method?**
    a. The father must have the condition and the mother must have the trait.
    b. The mother must have the condition and the father must have the trait.
    c. Both the father and mother must have either the sickle cell trait or condition.
    d. Either the father or mother can pass on the dominant gene to cause sickle cell.

35. **When caring for a baby with sickle cell anemia, the nurse recognizes what facts?**
    a. Pain experienced due to occlusion of blood flow and tissue ischemia is treated with cold packs initially.
    b. Blood cells are not transfused because the sickling will infect the new blood cells as well.
    c. Folic acid is used to release the blood cells and decrease clot formation and vessel blockage.
    d. Intravenous fluids are infused to maintain hydration and decrease the blood viscosity and clot formation.

36. **An infant who has hemophilia is likely to demonstrate what symptoms?**
    a. Formation of clots in the lower extremities
    b. Bone pain and anemia
    c. Bleeding after minimal trauma
    d. Fatigue due to poor blood cell production

37. **Thalassemia may be manifested through what symptoms?**
    a. Flushed face
    b. Large appetite
    c. Hyperactivity
    d. Headache

38. **What is the reason genetic testing is performed for family members when a baby is born with thalassemia?**
    a. It is important to discover the location of the gene for thalassemia so the infant can be cured.
    b. Siblings are at risk for being carriers and should have this information when planning a family.
    c. One parent must carry the dominant gene so the other parent may want to find a new partner so that the thalassemia gene will not be passed on.
    d. The mother can be shown the danger of passing thalassemia to her sons on the X-chromosome and the trait to her daughters.

39. **Which newborn would be at the highest risk for having Down syndrome?**
    a. The daughter of a woman who is 25 years old
    b. The newborn who is exposed to rubella
    c. The newborn who received high-caloric intake
    d. The son of a woman who is 43 years old

40. **If a pregnancy is unwanted, what likely options would a woman have?**
    a. Drink high volumes of water and disrupt the amnion development.
    b. Eat large amounts of folic acid to stimulate fetal rejection.
    c. Carry the baby the full term and place it up for adoption.
    d. Continued pregnancy is required if in or beyond the 2nd month of pregnancy.

41. **A prenatal history and physical reveal signs of infection with symptoms of flu. The nurse notes that the pregnant female enjoys eating pieces of raw steak with sauce. What condition might the nurse suspect and anticipate orders to treat?**
    a. Tiramisu
    b. Toxoplasmosis
    c. Cytomegalovirus
    d. Cystoplasmosis

42. **What does the "O" in the infection acronym TORCH represent?**
    a. Orchitis
    b. Oxyhemogobinemia
    c. Other infections
    d. Oncoginitis

43. **A woman in her first trimester of pregnancy complains of dyspareunia and pelvic pain over the past month. The nurse notes an elevated temperature and increased C-reactive protein levels. What procedure would the nurse prepare for?**
    a. An immediate abortion with suction
    b. Preoperative care for emergency surgery
    c. An ultrasound to determine the location of the fetus in the uterus
    d. Culture to find the cause of the pelvic inflammatory disease

44. **Women who test positive for gonorrhea are often automatically treated for what other STD?**
    a. Chlamydia
    b. Herpes
    c. Human papillomavirus
    d. Syphilis

45. **What is the most important reason that herpes should be diagnosed and treated as quickly as possible in a pregnant female?**
    a. The woman may pass the condition to her partner during sexual intercourse.
    b. Maternal death can occur if the vesicles rupture before they can be removed.
    c. Vitamin C therapy can be initiated quickly to eliminate the herpes virus.
    d. Newborn injury or death can be caused by genital tract herpes during birth.

46. **The primary care provider has diagnosed a 24-week pregnant female with syphilis. If the condition is passed to the fetus what would the nurse anticipate?**
    a. Instructing the family that the child will need lifelong care for control of the disease
    b. Monitoring the fetal development closely for possible intrauterine growth retardation
    c. Immediate infusion of antibiotic to the newborn after birth to reduce symptoms
    d. Counseling the parents as they grieve because the child has this incurable condition

47. **A pregnant woman presents at her prenatal visit with vaginal bleeding, and the examination reveals she has cervical dilation with an opening of the cervical os about the size of a dime. What condition would the nurse suspect?**
    a. Missed abortion
    b. Partial abortion
    c. Inevitable abortion
    d. Threatened abortion

48. **Which complaint would the nurse recognize as a sign of a serious complication in a 16-week pregnant female?**
    a. Small amounts of vaginal bleeding that is brown or bright red
    b. Nose-bleeding with swollen nasal passages and voice changes
    c. Breast and nipple enlargement with notable swelling of the veins
    d. Nausea and vomiting accompanied by hunger and intense cravings

49. **Which sign or symptom would be considered a presumptive sign of pregnancy?**
    a. Amenorrhea
    b. Ballottement
    c. Braxton-Hicks contractions
    d. Cervical changes

50. **What positive sign could be used with the greatest confidence to confirm that a woman is pregnant?**
    a. Quickening
    b. Fetal heart tones
    c. Cholasma
    d. Palpable fetal outline

51. **May is pregnant for the third time and has two living children, one that was born premature at 30 weeks. The nurse would describe her with what designation?**
    a. Gravida 1, para 2
    b. Gravida 3, para 2
    c. Gravida 1, para 3
    d. Gravida 3, para 1

52. **Why is it most important to determine both the maternal and paternal blood type and Rh factor?**
    a. If the mother is Rh positive and the father is Rh negative the fetus could cause a reaction that results in the mother becoming anemic.
    b. If the mother is Rh positive and the father is Rh positive the fetus could cause a reaction that results in the mother becoming anemic.
    c. If the mother is O negative and the father is B positive the fetus could cause a reaction that results in hemolysis in the fetus and anemia.
    d. If the mother is B positive and the father is O negative the fetus could cause a reaction that results in the mother becoming anemic.

53. **What associated condition would the nurse monitor for if a female in her second pregnancy is found to be Rh negative and the father is unknown?**
    a. Rubella
    b. Rubeola
    c. Erythroblastosis fetalis
    d. Erythematosis gravidarum

54. **At the prenatal visit Ms. Margis had a fundal height measurement of 29 centimeters. Using the McDonald method, what would the gestational age be?**
    a. 22 weeks.
    b. 29 weeks.
    c. The date of the last period is needed.
    d. Three months and 22 weeks.

55. **A female reporting for her first prenatal visit asks when she can expect to feel her baby moving. What would be the most accurate response?**
    a. "The baby should move before you finish your fourth month."
    b. "Relax, your baby won't move until you are at least 25 weeks."
    c. "When you are at about 20 weeks you might feel movement."
    d. "We need to know if your baby is not moving by your third month."

56. **In fetal circulation, how does blood entering the right side of the heart move to the left side of the heart? Blood flows in what direction?**
    a. From the right heart to the pulmonary artery to the lungs to the left side of the heart
    b. Through the patent ductus arteriosus to the left side of the heart
    c. Through a ventricular septal defect to the left side of the heart
    d. From the right atrium through the foramen ovale to the left side of the heart

57. **Identical twins would result from what pattern of conception?**
    a. Fraternal or dizygotic
    b. One ovum fertilized by two separate spermatozoa
    c. Two separate ova fertilized by one spermatozoa
    d. Maternal or monozygotic

58. **Fetal assessment reveals that a 28-week fetus has a length of 32 cm (C-R) and a weight of approximately 1100 g. What would the nurse conclude from these findings?**
    a. The fetus is longer than expected for this stage of development.
    b. Intrauterine growth restriction is evident from the findings.
    c. The findings support the risk for the fetus being SGA at birth.
    d. Preparations should be made for a post-term birth for this fetus.

59. **The nurse notes that an α-fetoprotein serum level report indicates a high level and would suspect that the newborn may reveal what condition at birth?**
    a. ABO incompatibility
    b. Gastroschisis
    c. Encephalitis
    d. Fetoproteinuria

60. **In explaining Down syndrome to parents, the nurse would include what information?**
    a. The underlying genetic defect is a missing trisomy 21 chromosome.
    b. The condition is not likely to cause any lasting effect on the child.
    c. Trisomy 21 is the most common condition and results in mental retardation of varying degrees.
    d. The degree of mental retardation in Turner (XO) females is generally severe and the child remains dependent on family.

61. **An infant is born at 37¹/₂ weeks with a weight of 3200 g. The newborn would be considered to be in what category?**
    a. Small for gestational age
    b. Large for gestational age
    c. Appropriate for gestational age
    d. Premature with intrauterine growth restriction
    e. Macrosomic with postmaturity

62. **A postmature newborn is likely to reveal what sign or symptom?**
    a. Polycythemia due to prolonged hypoxia
    b. Hydramnios due to polyuria of diabetes
    c. Heat sensitivity due to high metabolism
    d. Increased lanugo due to increased hair growth

63. **Baby boy Jennings was born at 35 weeks gestation with a birth weight of 2100 g. This infant would be considered which of the following?**
    a. High birth weight infant
    b. Post-term infant
    c. Small for gestational age
    d. Large for gestational age

64. **In preparation for childbirth what activities may be noted?**

    a. The father is instructed that he cannot enter the delivery room unless he is married to mother.

    b. A younger sibling is taught how to hold the scissors so he or she can cut the cord.

    c. The primary care provider decides what method of feeding will be used for the newborn.

    d. The expectant mother is told what to expect during the labor and delivery process.

65. **Which statement by an expectant mother would indicate additional teaching is needed regarding the purpose of the daily multivitamin prescribed for expectant mothers?**

    a. "The multivitamin will help me and my baby since I can't eat as much when I am nauseous."

    b. "The multivitamin will provide the folic acid that I need so that neural defects don't happen."

    c. "I should take the multivitamin daily so I have the necessary vitamins and minerals I need."

    d. "If I take the multivitamin each day I won't have to eat the vegetables and foods I don't like."

66. **What alternatives can expectant mothers use to taking antiemetics for nausea relief?**

    a. Vitamin E

    b. Vitamin D

    c. Vitamin B_6

    d. Vitamin K

67. **Vegetarians have special nutritional needs depending upon their regular intake. What would be appropriate prenatal teaching by the nurse for a woman who is a vegetarian?**

    a. Vegetarians may need additional vitamin D supplements to ensure adequate supply.

    b. Vegans must make sure to eat the vegetables that are low in calories to avoid excess weight gain.

    c. Lacto-ovo vegetarians must add protein supplements to ensure sufficient protein intake.

    d. Vegetarians who eat fish and shellfish should eat seafoods that are high in mercury.

68. **What is the primary reason binge and purge eating can be dangerous to the fetus?**

    a. Maternal self-esteem deficits can cause fetal distress.

    b. Excessive intake from binge eating can result in an LGA fetus.

    c. Intrauterine growth restriction of the fetus can occur from limited food intake.

    d. Purging will result in removal of essential vitamin D from the body.

69. **What types of substances are usually included in pica situations?**
    a. Wheat flour
    b. Corn bread
    c. Clay powder
    d. Dried potatoes

70. **What type of breakfast and lunch diet would be appropriate for a 14-year-old pregnant female?**
    a. Breakfast bar with lemon-lime soda; fish and chips with hush puppies and cola
    b. Orange juice and toast; spinach salad with ham and cheese and wheat crackers
    c. Donut and cappuccino; hamburger with extra mayonnaise, fries, and a milkshake
    d. Protein vitamin shake; Healthy Choice light pasta with chicken and diet soda

71. **What activity would be acceptable in planning activities for a pregnant female?**
    a. Kegel exercises in the sauna
    b. Jogging a half a mile each evening
    c. Walking for 30 minutes daily
    d. Swimming for 1 hour a day

72. **Back pain can be reduced through what action?**
    a. Sleeping
    b. Pelvic tilt
    c. Lying supine
    d. Sitting in a rocker

73. **What position could the pregnant mother choose for vaginal delivery of the baby?**
    a. The Lamaze position
    b. A 180-degree position
    c. A squatting position
    d. The fetal position

74. **An expectant mother indicates she wants to give birth in a bathtub. The nurse would provide information about what birthing method to this woman?**
    a. Dick-Read method
    b. Bradley method
    c. Lamaze method
    d. Leboyer method

75. **The nurse would expect to provide care for what condition if the expectant mother exhibited continuous nausea and vomiting due to the high hCG levels?**
    a. Hyperemesis gravidarum
    b. Acute placenta previa
    c. Abruption placenta
    d. Ectopic pregnancy

76. **If an expectant woman is exhibiting hypertension, headache, decreased level of consciousness and proteinuria at 4+ level, and hyperreflexia with intermittent seizures, the nurse should note that the woman is showing signs of what condition?**
    a. Mild preeclampsia
    b. Gestational hypertension
    c. HELLP
    d. Eclampsia

77. **Which symptoms would suggest that a pregnant female may have an ectopic pregnancy that has ruptured?**
    a. An elevated serum hCG level
    b. A decreased blood pressure
    c. An elevated progesterone level
    d. No fetal activity by week 4

78. **What statement is accurate regarding premature rupture of membranes?**
    a. Digital examination should be performed every 2 hours to assess membrane status.
    b. Speculum examination reveals a vaginal fluid that tests positive by nitrazine paper test.
    c. Corticosteroids are given to restore membrane stability and repair the rupture.
    d. If fetal lungs are not mature a cesarean delivery is performed and respiratory support is provided.

79. **The nurse should prepare for what treatment of a woman in preterm labor?**
    a. Tocolytics
    b. Oxytocin
    c. Thyroxine
    d. Glycogen

80. **Which mother should the nurse watch most closely for placenta previa?**
    a. Mrs. Parker, who is a 22-year-old woman of European race
    b. Mrs, Barfield, age 28, who is a nullipara unmarried female
    c. Miss Dennis, who is having a second cesarean birth
    d. Mrs. Taylor, a 30-year-old in her first pregnancy

81. **Mrs. Daily has been diagnosed with complete placenta previa and is having continued vaginal bleeding with a 36-week fetus. What nursing care would be appropriate?**
    a. Prepare for vaginal birth when the fetus is 38 weeks.
    b. Insert an IV into Mrs. Daily for induction of labor.
    c. Perform a vaginal examination to check for cervical dilation.
    d. Maintain strict bed rest for a week or longer, if possible.

82. **What treatment may be required for a woman with abruptio placenta?**
    a. Delivery of the fetus through cesarean delivery if fetal distress is noted
    b. Delivery of the fetus by cesarean birth if DIC is present
    c. Administration of immunoglobulin to decrease placental rupture
    d. Administration of glucose infusions to promote fetal lung maturity

83. **What assessment finding would indicate the presence of DIC?**
    a. Platelet count is increased.
    b. Fibrinogen levels are elevated.
    c. Extremities are flushed red.
    d. Prothrombin time is prolonged.

84. **A night snack with protein and carbohydrate is provided to an expectant mother with gestational diabetes to prevent what condition?**
    a. Hypoglycemia
    b. Preeclampsia
    c. Hypertension
    d. Hydramnios

85. **What signs of shock would the nurse expect to see on assessment of Mrs. Jones about 3 hours postdelivery?**
    a. Increase in diastolic blood pressure >10 mm Hg
    b. A pulse rate 10% below Mrs. Jones' baseline
    c. Rapid respirations
    d. Flushed face

86. **What is a sign of maternal distress during labor?**
    a. More intense and more frequent uterine contractions
    b. Uterine relaxation between 50-second contractions
    c. Heart rate of 150 to 180 beats per minute during labor
    d. Reports of needing to have a bowel movement

87. **Immobility, particularly after cesarean birth surgery, can result in which most potentially life-threatening complication?**
    a. Urinary stasis
    b. Deep vein thrombosis
    c. Pressure ulcer
    d. Muscle atrophy

88. **A woman who was diagnosed with gestational diabetes mellitus tells you she is prepared to take insulin injections for the rest of her life. What is your best response?**
    a. "You'll need to balance your diet with appropriate amounts of insulin."
    b. "It is good that you are prepared to deal with your disorder."
    c. "You will require additional insulin in addition to an oral antiglycemic agent since your diabetes will be more difficult to control."
    d. "You will recover following pregnancy; however, you are a risk for developing Type II diabetes mellitus later in life."

89. **Baby girl LeeAnn is born with Apgar scores of 5 and 7. The infant is experiencing respiratory difficulty. What would the nurse's immediate action for this infant be?**
   a. Establish an adequate circulatory pattern within 2 minutes.
   b. Clear the airway and establish respirations in 2 minutes.
   c. Prevent respiratory distress syndrome.
   d. Obtain the oxygen concentration in the circulating blood.

90. **What symptom would suggest a postpartal complication?**
   a. Lochia rubra 12 hours after birth
   b. Temperature of 38°C (100.4°F) or less
   c. Blood loss of less than 12 ounces in 24 hours
   d. 16 to 20 sanitary pads saturated in 24 hours

91. **The physician determines that Mrs. Jones is hemorrhaging from uterine atony. What would the nurse expect to administer?**
   a. Apresoline
   b. Zaroxyln
   c. Methergine
   d. Proventil

92. **What is an appropriate measure in caring for a client who has experienced a fourth-degree laceration of the perineum?**
   a. Encourage her to douche at least once a week to reduce organisms that may come in contact with the perineal area.
   b. Administer analgesic rectal suppositories to promote comfort.
   c. Encourage fluid intake and foods high in fiber to prevent hard stool.
   d. Administer an enema when necessary to prevent constipation.

93. **Baby girl Lathasa was born large for gestational age. After being delivered vaginally, what should this infant be carefully assessed for?**
   a. Increased intracranial pressure
   b. Hyperthermia
   c. Decreased red blood cell levels (anemia)
   d. Hyperglycemia

94. **A patient being treated for galactosemia is concerned that her son still vomits and has diarrhea although she stopped giving him milk. What is your best response?**
   a. "He likely has a viral infection."
   b. "Is he eating cakes, cookies, or pies?"
   c. "You have probably forgotten something."
   d. "Is he drinking soda?"

95. **A parent whose baby was born at 43 weeks gestation tells you that her son's cheek twitches every time she kisses him on the cheek. What is your best response?**
    a. "This is a muscle spasm and a sign of hyperglycemia, which occurs with LGA infants. I'll notify the health care provider immediately."
    b. "This is a sign of hyperviscosity, which occurs sometimes with LGA infants. I'll notify the health care provider immediately."
    c. "This is a muscle spasm and a sign of low calcium, which occurs sometimes with LGA infants. I'll notify the health care provider immediately."
    d. "This is the Chvostek's sign, which occurs sometimes with LGA infants after birth. I'll notify the health care provider immediately."

96. **What information listed below would support a newborn who is suspected of having coarctation of the aorta?**
    a. Cyanosis of the upper extremities
    b. Bulging carotid arteries
    c. Cool arms and no visible blood vessels
    d. Weak or absent femoral pulses

97. **A new nurse is about to palpate a newborn who has Wilms tumor. What is your best response?**
    a. "Observe the site before palpating."
    b. "Do not palpate the site of the tumor."
    c. "Always explain the procedure to the patient."
    d. "Review the disorder before visiting the patient."

98. **Baby Alice was born 2 days ago and now presents with poor feeding, fatigue, dyspnea, and a murmur. She is diagnosed with a patent ductus arteriosus. How is the alteration described?**
    a. Increased cardiac output
    b. Right-to-left shunt
    c. Left-to-right shunt
    d. Increased systemic blood flow

99. **By 8 hours of age, Charlie presents with a murmur and cyanosis. An echocardiogram reveals that the valve between the right atrium and right ventricle failed to develop and little blood flows between the two structures of the heart. What is this abnormality called?**
    a. Valvular regurgitation
    b. Mitral valve stenosis
    c. Tricuspid valve atresia
    d. Valvular transposition

100. A newborn baby is severely cyanotic. The ECG reveals transposition of the great arteries. Which of the following occurs with this defect?

a. The tricuspid is in the left ventricle.
b. The aorta leaves the right ventricle.
c. The pulmonary artery leaves the right atria.
d. An atrial septal defect closes with respirations.

ANSWERS

1. b	2. d	3. b	4. d
5. b	6. b	7. b	8. a
9. b	10. c	11. a	12. c
13. c	14. a	15. a	16. a
17. b	18. d	19. a	20. b
21. a	22. b	23. b	24. c
25. b	26. a	27. c	28. a
29. c	30. a	31. b	32. d
33. c	34. c	35. d	36. c
37. d	38. b	39. d	40. c
41. b	42. c	43. d	44. a
45. d	46. b	47. c	48. a
49. a	50. b	51. b	52. c
53. c	54. b	55. c	56. d
57. d	58. a	59. b	60. c
61. c	62. a	63. c	64. d
65. c	66. c	67. a	68. c
69. c	70. b	71. c	72. b
73. c	74. d	75. a	76. d
77. b	78. b	79. a	80. c
81. d	82. a	83. d	84. a
85. c	86. c	87. b	88. d
89. b	90. d	91. c	92. c
93. a	94. b	95. c	96. d
97. b	98. c	99. c	100. b

Index

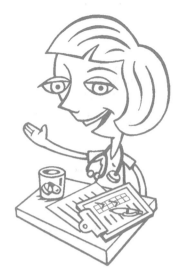

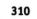